The Complete Guide to Holistic Health

Unlocking the Secrets of Biopsychosocial Wellness for Lasting Well-being

Conceived by:

Dr. Vladimir Friedman and Dr. Bob Davis

Published by: International Publications Media Group (IPMG)

Editor: Francois Nana Wilson

Dr. Vladimir Friedman conceived the necessity and guiding purpose of this book. A Doctor of Chiropractic Medicine with full-year postgraduate studies as a Certified Chiropractic Sports Physician, Certified Clinical Nutritionist, and certified practitioner of Electrodiagnostic Studies, Vlad has been a personal trainer and now is owner-therapist of Accelerated Care Chiropractic in Midtown Manhattan. Driven by a professional need to offer holistic therapy, Vlad has earned over 30 two-day post-grad certifications and over 50 lifetime certifications including EMT, first aid and safety, and lifeguarding.

Dr. Bob Davis, content supervisor, writing coach, and editor of this book, is a Ph. D. in Nineteenth-Century British Literature who taught university English for almost 40 years, principally at Clark University in MA and at NYU, where for 12 years he created, directed, and instructed a four-course program of expository prose for graduate students in the 22 majors of the Professional Studies Program. His published work includes *Your Writing Well: Common-Sense Strategies and Logic-Based Skills, in 15 Essays for the 21st Century,* instructor manuals for five college-level reading and writing anthologies, along with two volumes of literary criticism, style-diverse nonacademic prose, and poetry. As a freelance editor and language consultant for corporate and individual clients, Bob has been Copy-Chief for AOL Digital City New York, has development- and copy-edited over twenty volumes of literature for Houghton Mifflin's New Riverside Editions, edited online for The College Board and Pearson, and also edited for magazines, advertising agencies, architectural builders, and philanthropic foundations.

Luke Bongiorno, graduate of the University of Melbourne, Australia, is Director of the North American Neuro-Orthopaedic Institute

(Noigroup) in New York City and, previously, was co- founder of New York Sports Medicine. Recognized as one of the most prominent physical therapists in NYC, Luke not only is affiliated with the clinical education programs of Columbia University and Touro College and serves as a consultant with the NBA League, but also is internationally recognized for his treatment of professional and Olympic athletes and performing arts and dance company members, and for his consulting with professional European soccer teams.

Alex Cooksey, a Princeton graduate of East Asian Studies having recently changed his professional focus to computer software, was founder and trainer of Coaching with Cooksey in New Jersey, where he coached clients to achieve health and fitness goals through fully individualized exercise programming and a collaborative approach to value-based progressive behavior change.

Dr. Rob Curran, D.C. and EMT, is the Injury Prevention Coordinator/ Department of Trauma Surgery at New York Presbyterian/Weill Cornell Medical Center. In addition to his being the New York City Chapter Coordinator of the Sudden Cardiac Arrest Association and his providing extensive community service organization and instruction, he is or has been an adjunct faculty member and lecturer at seven colleges and universities throughout greater New York City.

Sharon Dominguez, an acupuncturist and founder of Ki Element Theory, is a Roku (6th) Dan ranked Aikido instructor, practitioner of Kototama Life Medicine, integrated strategist for structural, internal, and behavioral wellness, herbalist, non-denominational minister performing weddings and other important rituals, past stone and design specialist for high-end fashion jewelry, and flute player. She is the president of the board of the school New York Aikikai and a senior delegate with the International Aikido Federation in the Gender Balance Working Group. She teaches multi-styled meditation, classes both online and in person, including Kototama sound practice.

Dr. Marisa Galisteo, former Professor of Chemistry at U de Granada in Spain, biomedical research scientist at MIT and NYU Medical Center, and founder of Scientists as Leaders Training Co., is now a holistic practitioner integrating Energy Medicine ("The Energy Codes®"), Sound Healing, and The Sophia Code® in her Gentle Yoga offerings. An eternal student, she continues to explore what are the most effective ways to embody one's Higher Self, since this is key to better health, and she integrates them into her offerings, whether through Gentle Yoga, Sound Healing Circles or Sophia Circle Journeys™. She can be reached at marisa@marisagalisteo.com

Greg Grube's background includes swimming and diving, yoga instruction, and an individualized Pilates apprenticeship with Collette Stewart following the completion of his degree in dance from the University of Wisconsin, Madison; he also has a double-major B.A. in English and art history from UDelaware. While pursuing dance professionally, Greg gathered additional certifications from Eric Franklin (Level I and Level II) and a year-long professional dance program under the direction of Steve Paxton, a leading figure in the contemporary dance world. Already with over 1000 hours of training relevant to Pilates, Greg continues to explore and to study his interests in anatomy, biomechanics, functional movement, and somatic restoration.

Hicham Haouzi, 1988 Moroccan Olympic Taekwando team member and also gold medal Muay Thai winner in The Netherlands and twice in the U.S., is a Life and Personal Coach with over 20 years' experience at Equinox, where he's received a Lifetime Achievement Award and was cofounder of the first Equinox Games. Now, Hicham is General Manager of Hudson Yards' Equinox E Training Studios in Manhattan, the most elite coaching platform offered by Equinox; having designed that studio, Hicham also owns and runs HASTO Home Gyms.

Dr. Lanae Mullane brings a wealth of knowledge and expertise to her private practice in California. As the second naturopathic doctor to complete a residency with a focus on rheumatology, Dr. Mullane utilizes over a decade of clinical experience and a meticulous blend of biochemistry, nutraceuticals, nutrition, behavioral change, and comprehensive medical history to craft truly personalized experiences for each patient. Dr. Mullane delves into the intricacies of holistic health, offering a profound journey toward optimal well-being and resilience.

Maria Santoro, LMT, CSCS, ART, is a licensed massage therapist, movement therapist, and herbalist in New York City. Maria's approach is to provide treatment integrating both Western and Eastern techniques that are specific to each individual's physical, emotional, social, and spiritual well-being. Holding a degree in massage therapy from the Swedish Institute in New York City, Maria is trained in Swedish, Shiatsu, Thai, Reiki, Reflexology, Cranio-Sacral, myofascial release, structural integration, medical, sports, deep tissue massage, and active release technique (ART). Having completed advanced studies in physical anthropology, movement science, and rehabilitation, Maria provides therapy for neurological disorders in hospitals, rehabilitation facilities, and assisted living facilities. She is a NADA (National Acupuncture Detoxification Association) practitioner providing ear acupuncture, beads and seeds for addiction, stress, and trauma. She volunteers at NY-HRE, a harm reduction-based program in East Harlem one day a week. While living abroad in Asia, Maria studied Thai massage at Wat Pho School of Thai Massage in Bangkok and Medical Thai Massage with Nipha Sangkhwai. In Korea, Maria earned a 1st Dan Black Belt in Taekwondo. She is also a dedicated yoga practitioner, having studied Iyengar yoga in Pune, India and holding a certificate from ISTHA (Integrated Science of Hatha, Tantra and Ayurveda) in New York City. Some of her respected teachers are John Barnes, Dr. Michael Leahy, and Shiatsu master Ohashi. Maria is currently completing her second year of plant medicine at The Gaia School of Healing in Vermont. In addition to her passion for bodywork, movement, and herbal studies, Maria is a Japanese Zen Buddhism practitioner. Her devotion to her practice has allowed her to deepen her insight and mindfulness and thus to embrace each person she encounters with compassionate care. You can reach Maria by emailing her at msantoro144@gmail.com.

Nicole Visnic MS, CCN, CNS®
Niccle@analyticalnutrition.com
https://analyticalnutrition.com/ ▪
https://www.lifespanmedicine.com/
Nicole Visnic is a seasoned clinician with a proven track record of success. She has helped thousands of clients achieve their health goals through personalized nutrition and client-centered care. She specializes in conditions like chronic fatigue and functional gastrointestinal disorders. Nicole is the Director of Nutrition at LifeSpan medicine in Santa Monica, CA. She is also the founder of Analytical Nutrition. Nicole

earned her Master's Degree from the University of Bridgeport in Human Nutrition. She is a Certified Clinical Nutritionist (CCN) and a Certified Nutrition Specialist (CNS®).

Sam Visnic, CMT, is one of the nation's leading practitioners working to solve the complexities of chronic pain. Owner and Director of Release Muscle Therapy in Temecula, CA, and author of the e-book *Why Didn't My Doctor Tell Me That?*, Sam has studied dozens of methodologies for uncovering the root cause of aches and pains, including pain science, hands-on soft tissue massage techniques, myofascial release, and coaching movement.

TABLE OF CONTENTS

INTRODUCTION
Dr. Bob Davis

All of this book's fourteen authors—doctors, physical and massage therapists, fitness trainers—steadfastly believe and practice that wellness of the human body is the multifaceted result of physical, physiological, psychological, emotional, spiritual, and sociocultural factors, and that the human body and the brain with mind must be thought of as a holistic system of convergent functions and interconnections. Each participating writer acknowledges having been a specialist whose specialized education and applied practice to some extent determined—and on occasion limited—her or his professional destiny. Yet as these wellness experts' expertise developed within the restrictions of their specializations, they discovered their need to search beyond established boundaries of their standardized normal knowledge and to lift the lid off their boxed understandings. It wasn't enough for these masters to learn from only their specialized degree or degrees; therefore, reaching out, they borrowed from other ways and means of learning about wellness, from alternative practices, from theoretical and applied possibilities beyond but nonetheless compatible within the range of their specialty. In effect, all writers of this book integrated into their specializations other harmonious modes for wellness in an attempt to promote a more holistic health for their clients.

In "Towards a Definition of Holism," Joshua Freeman explains holistic health or wellness as "the ability to use a biopsychosocial model [George L. Engel's term] taking into account cultural and existential dimensions"; healers and health- promoters, Freeman continues, must acknowledge "that everything affects health [and] we must understand and honour the whole, in each of its parts and with the synergies that are created as they act together" (155). Holistic wellness therefore also must consider a patient's and client's day-to day lifestyle choices, routines and habits, emotional support systems and how they influence health, and the effects of all environmental and institutional contexts; thus, the well-being and total health of the body becomes inseparable from the brain's mind or psyche itself, while body and mind are influenced by external stimuli. This book uses the term "biopsychosocial" to indicate holistic wellness.

Our emphasis on holism—on integrating parts (at first, sometimes seemingly dissimilar parts) that add up to larger conceptual wholes—signifies a growing trend in human intellectual history's evolution of consciousness, how consciousness operates, and how it collectively imposes mental energy on material existence. For about the past 450 years, since the Renaissance and the birth of the scientific method, the "Newtonian paradigm" has been Westerners' rigorous intellectual model for thinking, perceiving the world, and validating facts and truths. Standard inquiry and analysis have been presupposed and informed by strict material empiricism interested in analyzing matter into single (atomistic) visible parts—sightings microscopic, observable to human eyes, and telescopic. Unchanging, Newton's "clockwork universe" was a non-evolutionary machine constructed by the Great Clockmaker, God, Who gave humans reason (so said the eighteenth- century Age of Reason or Enlightenment) to aid in deconstructing the material world into its fully knowable parts and, with physics, to discern their mechanistic interactions. Only slowly has the Newtonian paradigm yielded to concepts of evolution and everlasting change within the material world. In stages, Western thought has abandoned belief in the mechanical fixity of all living existence and appreciated, correctly, the interrelated, ever-weaving processes of energy contained by the material parts of our organic universe and solar system, planet Earth, and Her plants and animals.

With the aid of computers and the Internet, and with an increased understanding of benefits derived from an escalating focus on theoretical and factual interrelatability, humans have been shifting intellectually to convergent thinking, to a mode of integrative, academically interdisciplinary thought that joins parts into newly formed and understandable wholes. Recurring descriptors throughout this book on holistic or biopsychosocial wellness, "integrated" and "comprehensive" are explained in Josep Galliea's article "Integral Thinking," which "argues about the need to use a new modality of thinking, defined as integral thinking. . . . a kind of thinking that is holistic but also has span and profundity. . . . the kind of thinking appropriated to the contemporary need to think integrally in science, culture, professions, and arts or about the evolution of personal consciousness. It's useful also to be applied in the diverse professional fields, especially when comprehensive approaches are needed" (http://www.integralworld.net/gallifa4. html).

The seeds for this new mode of thought were planted slightly more than two centuries ago in the fertile soil of Western philosophy and art, and botanical and geological science, and today have begun to flower in all fields of human intellectual consideration, physics included. When applied to our lives and our world, convergent thinking merges interplaying ideas whose overlaps and synergies yield broader vision, deeper insight, and more meaningful foresight which, when applied to human existence, are intellectually greater than the sum of their parts and therefore are moving human consciousness upward, frequently raising it and us above the material limitations of our preceding paradigm. Convergence emergence is an unstoppable force of collective mental energy promoting greater sapience in *homo sapiens*, a truth evidenced in this book and in all that this book adds up to. One can say that whereas the Newtonian paradigm's accumulation of specialized knowledge has made us smarter about the world's material parts in isolation, the increased convergence of that smart knowledge—through integration and synthesis, through comprehensive and holistic thinking—is making us potentially wiser with the wholes which those parts add up to. An obvious example of convergent thinking backed by proof is humans' recent attention to the ecology and ecosystems of planet Earth, also a living body whose large-scale wellness depends on the collective small-scale biopsychosocial health of humans. Presently, neither our planet nor its population of people is commendably well. We're only beginning to apply and enact our new, holistic understandings wisely, sapiently.

Aiming its convergent ideas and comprehensive approaches to the field of integrated human health or holistic wellness, this book is purposed towards readers' biopsychosocial self-supervision, with practical truths providing knowledge and applicable tools with which all people can coach, repair, restore, develop, and maintain their biopsychosocial well-being. Idealism governs this book's intentions, not only because human biopsychosocial wellness is attainable to so many of our readers through careful self-assistance, but also because human wellness as a means for eliminating stress, promoting wisdom, and attaining peace can lead to larger holistic wellness for our societies and our planet.

Helping to explain the practical value of *The Complete Guide to Holistic Health* is the unifying premise of David Epstein's 2019 *Range: Why Generalists Triumph in a Specialized World*. Epstein argues that in most fields—especially those that are complex and unpredictable—generalists, not specialists, are better prepared to excel. People who think broadly and embrace diverse experiences and perspectives have the kind of sophisticated smarts—the wiser knowledge or sapience—that increasingly will help them to adapt and thrive in our dynamically changing twenty-first century worlds of business, technology, science, and medicine, among other professional pursuits. Creating an antibiotic vaccine against Covid-19 required a new range of convergent thinking, required "applying original thinking across domains" (Kapoor), "collaborative efforts across sectors of society" (Felter), and, for research, "identifying points of integration within a sequential convergent design using text mining to manage large data volumes and studying complex phenomena" (Poth). Already becoming increasingly collaborative and convergent, those worlds and their systems are de-emphasizing what Epstein characterizes as specialization's short-sighted thinking and instead are emphasizing broader, more integrated comprehensive perspectives that result in innovations created from multifaceted synergies. Such is the focused range in the reports by all authors of this book, themselves eclectic generalists even when labeled as specialists.

To more fully inform our understanding of integrative holism, let's set aside a few pages here to explore the limitations of specialization. Of course, first we gratefully must appreciate that Western medicine and knowledge of the human body have made notable educational and practical progress in specialist disciplines, and that specialist research and practice have led to diagnoses, preventions, treatments, and cures for specific diseases, illnesses, bodily ailments, injuries, and impairments. But specialism by its nature, and by Western institutional habit, works in isolation and still too often is unaware of or neglects the broader causes and fuller implications—the holistic range—of those aforementioned problem diseases, illnesses, and ailments. "Medical mistakes are far too common because each specialist is treating (or more likely over-treating) her own pet organ," says Dr. Allen Frances, Professor Emeritus of Psychiatry and former Chair at Duke University. "No one is considering the whole patient to organize a global, integrated, safe, and effective treatment plan." The patient as a whole is neglected, Frances continues, because "Unfortunately, doctors no longer know their patients. GPs [General Practitioners] are overworked, underpaid, and must shuttle patients in and out of the office . . . . Specialists tend to treat the test, not the patient, and earn their living doing procedures that often are unnecessary." Since 1961, the number of GPs in America has declined by one third, while specialization obviously has increased proportionally. Further problems with this trend are that "Specialty dominated practice also leads to inadequate preventive health services, late detection of diseases, and difficulty managing common chronic conditions such as obesity, diabetes, hypertension, and heart disease." In this context, writers of *The Complete Guide to Holistic Health* intend to serve also as a preventive health service.

As does this book, Frances argues for an educational holism in which, among other institutionalized requirements, "Medical school testing should be *comprehensive and integrated* [my emphasis], instead of the current common practice of administering exams based on discipline." Lacking a comprehensive overview of the patient, current medical specialism shows how "The doctor/patient relationship has lost its healing power. Doctors are too busy doing the wrong things. Patients have been reduced to a collection of lab test results." The purpose of good doctoring, therapy, and physical training for wellness and health care is a cultural necessity and ethical imperative, not primarily the bolstering of institutions' financial well-being, a trend whose origin in America, Frances explains, is rooted in the Flexner medical reforms of 1910 which despite their high medical standards advanced "a flaw that now haunts and distorts medical education and practice throughout the world." This flaw, based originally on Johns Hopkins University's "great emphasis on departmental specialization and research productivity," has become the model for achieving the financial goals of attracting the most research dollars and of producing the most clinical revenue by doing costly medical and surgical procedures. Conversely, "Primary care teaching and practice has always been deeply devalued by medical centers," Frances concludes, "because it does neither [kind of financial gain advocacy]." Money still talks, and talks loud, even if greater human wellness is being cumulatively silenced. Frances' article's subtitle sums this up: We should be "Putting the patient, not the procedure, in the center of medical care."

Nearly 20 years ago, the authors of "Integrative Medicine: Bringing Medicine Back to Its Roots" noted the irony that, "just when decades of biomedical research are beginning to pay miraculous dividends, public confidence in the medical establishment is eroding" because of "the gap between what many conventional health care providers deliver and what the public wants and needs" (395). Essentially, according to that article, "a public need for holism in medicine is clashing with the industry's most fundamental, reductionist ways," reductionism being the medical industry's emphases on specialization. Dr. Snyderman et al. highlight the need for conventionalized integrative medicine, agreeing with its "calls for restoration of the focus of medicine on health and healings and emphasi[s on] the centrality of the patient-physician relationship" (Snyderman, 396).

Granted, increased numbers of Americans recently have gained access to networks of specialists from top-tier hospitals, comprehensive health care systems, and medical concierge referral services or alliances, specialists working under the same healthcare umbrella and consequently doing better both to improve patients' wellness through teamwork and to upgrade technology for transferring test results and prescriptions. But complementary healthcare systems are principally urban and academic, remain time-consuming and often prohibitively expensive, and still don't eliminate the inherent flaw associated with specialization: its financially skewed perspectives on healthcare.

The disadvantages of specialization's reductionist approaches are best understood when we examine "multimorbidity," the ugly-named condition of patients with multiple chronic diseases, a population of patients "quickly becoming the norm" (*The Atlantic*). A 2014 study of 60,000 Americans found that 59.6% or three- fifths were typed multimorbid (https://www.jabfm.org/ content/31/4/503). Given the population density of multimorbidity, we should be concerned about how specialization functions when we further learn that

> Not only do multimorbid patients receive suboptimal care, but the unnecessary hospitalizations, redundant tests, and disjointed care they receive put disproportionate pressure on our health system. . . . specialists rarely know how the treatment they administer interacts with other concurrent treatments (The Atlantic).

What we learn from our country's medical and therapeutic emphasis on specialization is that a fragmented, piecemeal approach to wellness has not made and never will contribute to making us a healthy nation. "Best Healthcare in the World Population 2020" offers global statistics that use evaluative criteria set by the World Health Organization. Countries having universal healthcare rank notably high in this study; the United States ranks 37th, between Costa Rica and Slovinia, and by global standards looks dismally deprived of effective national medical services and health care, a fact whose roots obviously extend beyond but nonetheless include specialization.

The many contributing causes leading to Americans' unfortunate lack of wellness are being studied and addressed but aren't yet changing in ways leading to improving America's collective wellness. Added to the problems within American health care and its widespread financial inaccessibility are four other contributing deterrents to our national wellness: medication errors and American overuse of prescriptive drugs; unhealthful family habits and behaviors, notably harmful cultural patterns of food consumption and their consequent high levels of obesity and illness;[2]+[3] inherent social conditions promoting unhealthful norms; and inadequate public knowledge of and education programs for teaching wellness. Statistically, it's an obvious conclusion that the U. S. isn't a nation of healthy people, at least not relatively speaking: "Americans live shorter lives and experience more injuries and illnesses than people in other high-income countries. . . . This health disadvantage is particularly striking given the wealth and assets of the United States and the country's enormous level of per capita spending on health care, which far exceeds that of any other country" (National Research Council).

And from a cultural viewpoint it's easy to see that America's wellness is further sidetracked because too many people's brains are overstuffed with visual and verbal marketing that portrays and bespeaks the media's misleadingly idealized, usually unattainable standards for looks, bodies, and lifestyle, marketing that implies our insufficiencies

9

for not appearing like, measuring up to, and living those standards. Subliminal and conscious doubts about our looks, physical bodies, and lifestyle can—and for many people do—affect self-perception, which then becomes their reality; such reality can foster false beliefs about and goals for wellness. Further, this kind of value-laden vision promotes the misconception that attractively formed bodies necessarily indicate fitness or are equal to wellness and health; that, of course, is an empirical fallacy, as countless factors are involved in complete physical wellness, not just pumping iron in a fashionable gym, not just aerobic exercise on a sandy beach in the Hamptons or Malibu, not just stretchability and agility down a snowy slope in Aspen. Pretty frames very possibly obstruct our view of unseen problems that need to be attended to and cared for when wellness is our goal. Wellness is a multi-faceted construct best understood by holists, whose integrationist and broad-range or comprehensive thinking looks into the larger medical, anatomical, and practical pictures within which complete health exists. Moreover, optimal wellness is the result not only of a healthy body, but also of the well mind and intellect, emotions, psyche or spirit, and stressless interaction with society. Not judging a book by its cover, we must learn to inspect and respect its content and contexts, and to be confident that we author our own book wisely.

Given these national limitations and psychological misconceptions concerning wellness, *The Complete Guide to Holistic Health* is devoted to educating anybody anywhere who wants to improve her or his wellness and health. We offer preventive measures with which to avoid multimorbid complications—and strategies and practices for wellness that can modify or repair such complications. Here you'll find accessible explanations, enduring lessons, and reliable instructions from degreed and certified practitioners whose evolving professional research, scientifically validated learning, and personal ethics regarding the sensible preventions and prudent revitalizing strategies for wellness have enlightened them as holistic thinkers beyond the pale of reductive specialization. In their respective professional fields, all writers of this book have been ahead of the times, moving their practice towards a more integrated comprehensive approach to wellness; together, as a unit, their holism takes on new dimensionality, a deeper and broader overview and understanding of what makes us tick best. While some people may see holism and reductionism as opposites, this book will prove that there is overlap between the two, with room for each in the world of medicine, physical therapy, and fitness training. Holism does not seek to drive out reductionism or specialization; instead, it seeks to complement it by recognizing—and then converging—added pieces to the puzzle of wellness or added colors to the full spectrum of health.

The Covid-19 pandemic certainly has forced humans to puzzle out the implications of maintaining their own wellness and the complications from failing to do so, especially when unhealthful habits develop without our noticing. Commonly affected, many of us have experienced directly for ourselves or indirectly among family and friends the decline of physical health, breakdown of dependable psychological security, compromises to financial livelihood at home, collapses of business and industry around us, fragmenting of professional structures and systems, minimizing of interpersonal education, removal of cultural events, and in some instances even the fracturing of family. Undoubtedly a time of increased physical inactivity, psychological pressures, economic hardship, and social distancing, the Covid-19 pandemic has impacted—and has demanded restoration of—our individual and collective biopsychosocial wellness.

The varying kinds and degrees of biopsychosocial hardship are now behind us, but global frustration remains in our collective remembrance and informs our "new normal." Covid's imposed blackouts on all of the world at this decade's beginning remain as dark shadows from the residual consequences of psychological worry and fret—and the stress that comes with it all. For some people, bereavement has been a reality; for many others, isolation and its separations continue to loom larger than we might have expected. For everyone, fears of future uncertainties and deprivations, changes and adjustments have hit home. Indeterminacies of all kinds have imposed undue stress among many sectors of our society.

And what has this added up to? In one way, "Call it a . . . crisis of productivity, of will, of enthusiasm, of purpose," a crisis that "left many of us feeling like burned-out husks, dimwitted approximations of our once-productive selves" (Lyall). Clinically known as "behavioral anhedonia," this burned out, dimwitted feeling comes with people's inability to take pleasure in their activities, which in turn causes lethargy and lack of interest, which ultimately slackens their productivity. The less clinical but popular psychological term for this condition is "languishing," the opposite of flourishing, a lack of interest in what typically can bring joy.

Resilience against these kinds of psychological slumps has been difficult for many people to summon or to actualize, especially if one's body has been sequestered in relative isolation. Intensifying these psychological slumps, physical inactivity with its accompanying neuromuscular deconditioning has eroded many people's biological fitness during the pandemic. Sedentary habits aren't surprising when people have worked and lived exclusively from home in repetitive stationary positions, with movement bounded. And in many instances the national decline in activity and good health grew worse during the pandemic's first two or three months, when patients were unable to see their doctors, dentists, and other healthcare providers. Now, post-pandemic, patients with diseases and health problems other than Covid frequently report having experienced neglect, as human care redistributed to fight Covid has created not only an overload on doctors and other healthcare professionals, but also a disruption in the medical supply chain.

The Complete Guide to Holistic Health is timed to coincide with our nation's need to reactivate physically, reassert psychologically, reconnect socially (without neglecting still-needed sensible protocols), and self-educate as we review our biopsychosocial habits and behaviors. Wellness education and the self-practices learned from thorough, reliable instruction must become our routine self-expectation. Unfortunately, further downgrading America's standards for wellness is our nation's inadequate physical education institutionally, which in schools ought to be the foundation for people's understandings of wellness and maintaining personal health. Despite this, "An Analysis of Research on Student Health-Related Fitness Knowledge in K–16 Physical Education Programs" observes that

> Two major results [in its study] . . . are misconceptions about fitness and the lack of an adequate amount of human-related fitness (HRF) knowledge among students at all educational levels (i.e., elementary, secondary, and college). These results were essentially the same as those found more than 20 years ago, indicating a persistent deficiency in fitness education (Keating 333).

This contemporary article highlights the inadequacies not only of students' understanding of fitness, but of curricular content and physical educators' instruction—if school systems haven't already eliminated such instruction. Those inadequacies, for many of us, have been our inheritance.

So it's time for each of us to help ourself. But deciding on what's reliable information and practice isn't always easy and can be daunting amid trending fads, opposing views, and far too much unreliable online foolishness. How, then, do we separate the wheat from the chaff, the enduring facts from the trendy fads, the permanently proven from the provisionally experimental? This book already has done that for you, each of its authors offering reliable holistic help for everyone to learn what wellness is and how to accomplish it. Hope exists actively here in this book, where what you learn comes from reliably validated and scientifically replicated research, with instructive explanations and integrated holistic methods and tools to help yourself become a healthier, thus happier person.

The Complete Guide to Holistic Health's foundational principles add up to safe, advisable procedures for laying out your self-help paths to wellness and for guiding yourself towards self-maintenance. As do all ethically concerned doctors, therapists, and trainers, this book's authors recommend that you seek specialist help whenever a situation warrants special attention beyond what you can do on your own. That said, this book offers verified guidelines and strategies that will save you time, money, and needless physical and psychological aggravations and that will provide the proper building blocks to structure your future wellness and health programs: frequently our well-being is in our own hands, ours to do with as we see fit—long before professional medicine or therapy or training must intercede. Therefore, *The Complete Guide to Holistic Health's* intention is to offer instruction on the bodily, mental, and behavioral additions and modifications that will foster wellness for you, whatever your state of wellness presently may be. In effect, as self-helping instruction containing foundational biopsychosocial wellness principles, this book will assist readers with preventive, curative, and maintenance practices needed for being well and for well-being. Many of us know how Internet research about diagnoses and management of any physical condition can be dead-ended, or confusingly open-ended, and sometimes needlessly alarming to readers, whereas this book's discussions of assured behaviors and dependable practices provide controlled supervision throughout all wellness processes, with wellness developed naturally according to each individual's individual needs.

The Complete Guide to Holistic Health's begins with a chapter by Dr. Vladimir Friedman, who conceived its depth of purpose and breadth of investigation. Vlad maps and explains his eclectic personal and professional pursuit of biopsychosocial wellness, a journey whose visited destinations allow for a thorough theoretical and practical understanding of what biopsychosocial wellness means in general and therefore will mean specifically to each of you. The book then explores the enduringly valuable fundamentals or bottom-line necessities to consider when making biopsychosocial wellness one's own; no reader will be able to appreciate the meanings of wellness, to work self- helpfully towards it, and to live well without this fundamental knowledge. To undo your harmful personal traits and to create helpful ones, readers next will become acquainted with strategic skills and practices structured by behavioral conditioning to break bad habits and breed good ones before or during any wellness program. Just as behavior change can occur anytime in one's life, so too can anxiety and pain, and especially chronic pain lasting more than six months; these important topics are explored biopsychosocially by two of this book's experts, who scientifically explain the causes and effects of pain, and how and where to deal therapeutically with it. Following that are multiple discussions devoted to human resilience as maintained by proper nutrition, effective sleep, and stress management, subjects that will benefit all readers, as will our professional observations for people with orthopedic musculoskeletal injuries and in need of massage therapies in clinics or at home, through healing touch and self-massage. Throughout the book but principally in its final third are Eastern understandings and practices of wellness which meet and converge with those of the West, thus forming a global partnership for smart health that legitimizes *The Complete Guide to Holistic Health's* truly integrated comprehensive presentation. This book infuses Asian philosophical lessons and practices, including acupuncture, protocols and guides to live by for wellness, purification ceremonies, ways to mitigate sickness and to attain self-healing balances through body work, meditation, and sounds. Last but not least, biopsychosocial self-healing and wellness, and detailed guides for exercise, are viewed through the lenses of our experts with yoga, Pilates, and motion and exercise training for fitness. All of our physical training's techniques and tips promote athletic performance not only by identifying weakness in optimal stability and mobility, but also by improving fundamental movement capacities (FMC) of mobility, balance, coordination, stability, strength, power, speed if applicable, and endurance.

To attain genuine total wellness, people need guides whose wisdom-based knowledge is focused purposefully, reasoned comprehensively, and integrated patiently, not haphazard bits and pieces of scattered information fragmented throughout the public domain and in specialist tomes, or popularized by trendy, short-lived fads. This book's accessible outlook, with best-practice lessons from the West and the East, and informed by wellness holists writing about their holistic practices, is heightened and further unified by the "Index of Recurring Subjects" at its end. There, yet another source of holism exists, as readers will be able to create their own thorough overview of important subjects of interest or concern as treated by whichever writers of *The Complete Guide to Holistic Health* address them. If for example you're interested in "breathing," "enteric nervous system,"maybe "subconscious" or "voices, self-doubting," then under each of those headings you'll find a complete list of pagination leading you through a comprehensive understanding of those subjects from our writers' multiple and diverse but never contradictory points of view. Packed with opportunity, the Index will allow you to create in unity your own tracts for all subjects you'd like to discover more about. This book is devoted to facilitating and guaranteeing your self-education. Further, we hope *The Complete Guide to Holistic Health* will be useful to other wellness practitioners as a mindful spur to their already existing awareness of the theoretical and practical importance of integrated comprehensive wellness. Some of those practitioners already think convergently but need a catalyst to conjoin with similar thinkers, while other such practitioners may be just beginning to appreciate the functional imperatives of integrated comprehensive wellness and its biopsychosocial components. Whatever the kind and degree of this book's influence, its authors have been dedicated to establishing for public and peer awareness a consolidated multifaceted understanding of the next step or new wave in well-founded, properly practiced biopsychosocial wellness. Just as science historian Peter Watts' 2019 Convergence painstakingly details the theoretical and applied developmental overlaps and integrations among the biological and physical sciences from 1859 to the present, so *The Complete Guide to Holistic Health: Unlocking the Secrets of Biopsychosocial Wellness for Lasting Well-being* recognizes and explains the convergent modalities that already exist—even if not yet frequently observed and applied by professionals—in the scientific studies and practices of human wellness.

ENDNOTES

[1]Americans "live in a culture, say the experts [whom *Consumer Reports* consulted], encouraged by intense marketing by drug companies and an increasingly harried healthcare system that makes dashing off a prescription the easiest way to address a patient's concerns" (Carr). Wanting and receiving feel-better quick fixes and long-term remedies, we rely on healthcare practitioners to responsibly know about and to ethically administer our drugs; consequently, we're inclined to feel safe about consuming them. Due to this over-reliance on drugs coupled with our assumption of their safety and proper prescription, "The percentage of Americans taking more than five prescription medications has nearly tripled in the past 20 years, according to the Centers for Disease Control and Prevention"; Dr. Michael Hochman adds that unfortunately "The risk of adverse events increases exponentially after someone is on four or more medications" (Carr). This exponential increase happens more commonly when multimorbid patients have multiple specialists. It's fair to conclude that prescription drug misuse is prevalent in America. "The reasons for the high prevalence of prescription drug misuse vary by age, gender, and other factors," says the National Institute on Drug Abuse, "but likely include ease of access" (https://www.drugabuse.gov/publications/research-reports/misuse-prescription-drugs/what-scope-prescription-drug-misuse).

While it's true that "Prescription opioids, also known as prescription painkillers, have become a popular staple in medicine cabinets across the United States, resulting in devastating misuse, addiction and overdose" (Carr), we'd be naive to assume that full responsibility for inflated use of these drugs is attributable alone to bad decisions by patients. Ease of access to prescription drugs is attributable also to America's bedeviling pharma-drug production. A 2019 Drugwatch reported that "Prescription drug use is a global problem, and the U.S. is the world's biggest addict"; we consume 99% of the world's Vicodin, 80% of Percoset and OxyContin, and 60% of Dilaudid (Elkins). Since 1999, American deaths by overdose of prescribed painkillers have quadrupled; recent data show "The amount of harm stemming from inappropriate prescription medication is staggering. Almost 1.3 million people went to U.S. emergency rooms due to adverse drug effects in 2014, and about 124,000 died from those events. That's according to estimates based on data from the Centers for Disease Control and Prevention and the Food and Drug Administration" (Carr). More than 6.5 million people use prescription medication for non-medical reasons, which is more than cocaine, heroin, and hallucinogens combined. Further, overuse of antibiotics and antidepressants continues to skyrocket. And what has this added up to? "[T]he paths to high-quantity prescriptions and dependencies collided in the 21st century" (Elkins). And it's a proven fact that high-quantity prescriptions are further generated by a knowing collusion between pharma's drug manufacturing and many doctors' casually immoderate drug prescribing, yet another unfortunate fact contributing to increased abuse, addiction, and death.

Further, frequent medication errors both in hospitals and at pharmacies cause unnecessary illness and death in the United States. "Medical errors," occurring at multiple points in the prescription process at hospitals—for reasons as avoidable as indecipherable handwriting—"are considered the third leading cause of death in the United States" according to a 2016 Johns Hopkins study; "The American Association for Justice estimates that 440,000 errors resulting in death occur each year" (https://scartelli.com/pharmaceutical-errors/). Pharmaceutically, letters to state regulatory boards and interviews with *The New York Times* reveal that pharmacists at CVS, Rite Aid, and Walgreens, among other major drugstore chains, "described understaffed, chaotic workplaces and said it had become difficult to perform their jobs safely, putting the public at risk of medication errors." Seventeen years ago was the last comprehensive study of pharmaceutical medication errors, when "The Institute of Medicine estimated in 2006 that such mistakes harmed at least 1.5 million Americans each year" (*The New York Times Morning Brief*). Annually in the United States 7,000 to 9,000 people die as a result of a pharmacy medication error, and "The total cost of looking after patients with medication-associated errors exceeds $40 billion each year (Tariq). Additionally, hundreds of thousands of other patients experience but often do not report an adverse reaction or other complication related to a medication. And it's likely that the mishandling of meds has become worse, because "One of the major causes for medication errors is distraction. Nearly 75% of medication errors have been attributed to this cause" (Tariq); it follows that if a pharmaceutical workplace is "chaotic," just as most hospitals necessarily are, then errors of distraction are more likely to ensue. No statistics yet exist for Covid-occasioned prescriptive mishandlings, but the pandemic likely increased the chaos.

2+3Not altogether surprising, the relationship between easy access to and overconsumption of drugs is paralleled in Americans' easy access to and overconsumption of food, particularly unhealthful food at take-out restaurants. According to a December 2018 report, "Every day, more than 1 in 3 U.S. adults [84.8 million, or 37%] eat some type of restaurant fast food, according to a recent report from the National Center for Health Statistics" (*Safety Health*); this report reveals also that about the same percentage of children daily consume fast food. A major health concern, "Fast-food consumption has been associated with increased intake of calories, fat and sodium, which can lead to obesity, diabetes and other health issues, according to the researchers" (*Safety Health*); not unexpectedly, fast food is "low in several key nutrients that adult bodies need to flourish and that children's bodies need to grow" (*ABC Action News*). Exacerbating this trend of too many children eating too much unhealthful food, "American public schools have problems with putting out healthy meals" (Cheung). Supersizing ourselves, many Americans become obese. Obesity is defined as a person having a body mass index (BMI) of 30 and up. Measuring body fat as based on a weight to height ratio, the BMI includes three ascending Classes for obesity, with Class 3 having a BMI of 40 and over. The normal range for one's BMI is 18.5 to <24.9. People between a 25 and 30 BMI are classified as "overweight".

In most high-income countries, around two-thirds of adults are over-weight or obese. In the US, 70% are; worse, a 2018 article in *Our World in Data* notes that American obesity "nearly tripled between 1975 and 2016" (Ritchie). And every available article on obesity since the pandemic emphasizes that the trend of increased obesity continues. The October 2019 *World Population Review's* global rating of popu-lation obesity ranks the United States in 16th position, a ranking that included all age groups ("U.S. Obesity Rates"). Closer examination of this statistic shows that of the 15 countries with greater obesity, nine have a total population under 65,000 people, most of them living on tropical islands; another five countries are populated between 100,000 and 200,000, about the size of Dayton OH; and one, Kuwait, has slightly over four million people. Because all 15 more obese countries' populations total slightly over five million people, the 16th-place ranking of the U.S., which has over 330 million people, is deceptive; it misleadingly neglects to emphasize the widespread mass of obesity throughout our country. The pandemic's impact on consumers has increased global reliance on fast food, not curbed it. Nathaniel Ashby's study hypothesizes that the pandemic increased feelings of stress and anxiety that led and still leads to the emotional eating of unhealthy foods (Ashby). Skyrocketing grocery store prices sent consumers back to fast-food restaurants, now more convenient because of restarted drive-through and mobile pickup operations (Myers). And "It isn't just the price that makes fast food attractive. Parents are juggling working and looking after their kids who are spending more time at home. . . . These time-strapped Americans are turning to the convenience of take-out food, and many delivery services are soaring. Domino's reported that its US same-store sales . . . generated $240 million in net income - 30% higher than in 2019 (Dean). And fast-food convenience continues to increase technologically with app proliferation and the food-marketers' ability to connect with customers through automated ordering and payments.

WORKS CITED

ABC Action News, Lifestyle Section, "CDC report: 84.8 million U.S. adults consume fast food every day and other startling findings," Oct 03, 2018

American Cancer Society, Cancer Action Network, "Increasing and Improving Physical Education and Physical Activity in Schools: Benefits for Children's Health and Educational Outcomes" https://www.ightcancer.org/policy-resources/keeping-children healthyrecommendations-promoting-physical-education-and-physical

Ashby Nathaniel J. S. "The impact of the COVID-19 pandemic on unhealthy eating in populations with obesity." Obesity, 2020. doi:10.1002/oby.22940

Best Healthcare in the World Population 2020 (2019-10-24) from http://worldpopulationreview.com/countries/best-healthcare-in-the-world/

British Journal of General Practice. 2005; 55 (511): 154-155

Carr, Teresa, "Too Many Meds? America's Love Affair With Prescription Medication." Consumer Reports, August 3, 2017 https://www.consumerreports.org/prescription-drugs/too-many-medsamericas-love-affair-with-prescription-medication/

Cheung, Kylie, "How School Lunches Around the World Compare to America's." March2, 2016) https://archive.attn.com/stories/6085/school-lunches-around-worldcompared-to-the-united-states

Committee on Physical Activity and Physical Education in the School Environment; Food and Nutrition Board; Institute of Medicine, Educating the Student Body: Taking Physical Activity and Physical Education to School. Washington (DC): National Academies Press (US); 2013.

Introduction

Dean, Grace, Insider, **https://www.businessinsider.com/** american-kids-were-eating-more-fast-food-before-the-pandemic-2020-8).

Elkins, Chris, "Hooked on Pharmaceuticals: Prescription Drug Abuse in America." *Drugwatch*, May 17, 2019.

Epstein, David, *Range: Why Generalists Triumph in a Specialized World*, Riverhead Books, An imprint of Penguin Random House L.L.C., New York, NY, 2019

Felter, Claire, "A Guide to Global Covid-19 Vaccine Efforts." Council on Foreign Relations, October 2021. https://www.cfr.org/backgrounder/guide-global-covid-19-vaccine-**efforts** **https://** www.forbes.com/sites/benmidgley/2018/09/26/the-six-**reasons-thefitness-industry-is-booming/#16a8bb31506d.**

Frances, Allen, M.D., "We Have Too Many Specialists and Too Few General Practitioners," *Psychology Today*, Jan 21, 2016

--------"Patient-Centered Vs. Lab-Centered 'Personalized Medicine," Huffington Post Updated July 24, 2017

Freeman, Joshua, "Towards a Definition of Holism." *British Journal of General Practice, 2005* Feb 1; 55(511): 154-55

Galliea, Josep, "Integral Thinking." Integral World, Newsletter 812: November 30, 2019 http://www.integralworld.net

Griffiths, Sarah, "Bingeing on fast food leaves a scar etched in your DNA which is passed down to your children, study finds." *Daily Mirror*, 7 July, 2014.

Jones, Thomas C. and Betsy M. Chalfin, *From the Family Doctor to the Current   Disaster of Corporate Health Maintenance.* AuthorHouseUK, 2016.

Kapoor, Hansika and James C. Kaufman, "Meaning-Making Through Creativity during COVID-19." Frontiers in Psychology, 18 December 2020 **(https://doi.org/10.3389/fpsyg.2020.595990)**

Keating, Xiaofen Deng et al, "An Analysis of Research on Student Health-Related Fitness Knowledge in K–16 Physical Education Programs." Human *Kinetics Journals*, V. 28: Issue 3, 333-349.

Landhuis, Esther, "Your Immune System Is Made, Not Born." *Scientific American* January 29, 2015

Lyall, Sarah, "We Have All Hit a Wall." *The New York Times*, April 3, 2021. **https://www.nytimes.com/2021/04/03/business/pandemic burnoutproductivity.** html?campaign_id=9&emc=edit_nn_20210404&in-stance_id=28847&nl=themorning&regi_id=106975020&seg-ment_id=54857&te=1&userid=9ce00b47b37a6b7f1190627dae9e2fba

Miller, Kenneth. "Why Food Allergies Are Surging," *Leapsmag*, May 9, 2019.

Myers, Candice A. and Stephanie T. Broyles, "Fast Food Patronage and Obesity Prevalence During the COVID-19 Pandemic: An Alternative **https://doi.org/10.1002/oby.22993).**

National Research Council (US); Institute of Medicine (US), U.S. Health in International Perspective: Shorter Lives, Poorer Health. Washington (DC): National Academies Press (US); 2013.

Poth, Cheryl N. et. al, "Using Convergent Sequential Design for Rapid Complex Case Study Descriptions: Example of Public Health Briefings During the Onset of the COVID-19 Pandemic." **https://doi.org/10.1101/2020.11.11.20229393**

Ritchie, Hannah and Max Roser, "Obesity," Our World in Data, 2020 **https://ourworldindata.org/obesity**

Safety Health, Dec 6, 2018. "Nearly 37 percent of Americans regularly eat fast food, study shows"

Sawyer, Bradley and Daniel McDermott, "How do mortality rates in the U.S. compare to other countries?" Peterson-KFF Health System Tracker, February 14, 2019.

https://www.healthsystemtracker.org/chart-collection/mortality-rates-u-scompare-countries/

: 6/18/11, p. 26.

Simon, William E. Jr., "Physical education is key to longer, happier lives. Our kids and schools need more of it," USA Today, Dec 12, 2018 Snyderman, Ralph and Weil, Andrew T. "Integrative Medicine: Bringing Medicine Back to Its Roots." Archives of Internal Medicine. 2002. 62(4).

Tariq, Rahan A. and Yevgenia Sherbak, "Medication Errors," StatPearls

The New York Times Morning Brief, Friday, Jan 31, 2020.

https://www.nytimes.com/2020/01/31/briefing/president-trumpcorona-virus-brexit.html?te=1&nl=morning-briefing\
&emc=edit_NN_20200131&campaign_i d =9 & i n s t a n c e _ i d =1 5 628&segmen-tid=20853&user_id=9ce00b47b37a6b7f1190627dae9e2fba&regi_id= 10697502020200131

"U.S. Health in International Perspective: Shorter Lives, Poorer Health"

https:// www.ncbi.nlm.nih.gov/books/NBK154469/

"U.S. Obesity Rates Reach Historic Highs," Trust for America's Health, 2019

CHAPTER I

Why Biopsychosocial Wellness or Holistic Health?

Dr. Vladimir Friedman

Everyone wants the answers to pain-free optimal health and wellness, but are they ready for that commitment which those answers provide? Dedication is what makes or breaks clients' or patients' ability to succeed in anything, specifically achievements and outcomes in human performance and recovery. Being in the healthcare and fitness industry for over 25 years, I still find it incredibly difficult to guarantee results for any outcome. These days at gatherings, the initial introduction of who I am or what I professionally do usually triggers people's immediate hand-grab on my neck or low back and a reminder that they have been meaning to speak to someone like me. Daily questions arise in my clinical health care practice, Accelerated Care Chiropractic, and personal life about the best tools, systems, and strategies to ensure optimal wellness.

I am a practitioner who envisioned a book that would help guide the reader for best practices from some of the best individual doctors, therapists, coaches, and trainers. I recognized that all of these people, in different ways because of their specialties, share with me a passion for bringing to their specialization the best and widest-ranging complementary practices and tools to assure total wellness for their clients. And like me, all writers of this book recognize that as holists, or "jack- of-all trades and master of one," they know who can do better with certain

28

other aspects of wellness than they do. The most successful healthcare professionals understand their own best qualities but are most effective when they realize that other holists may be more advantageous for a client than themselves.

There are many times I am asked why I am so different from the other practitioners in my field, and unfortunately I do not have an answer other than I love the human body and how it functions, along with the humbling thank-you I receive when a patient's problem is resolved. My continual training and learning about my craft is what keeps me, I believe, ahead of the pack. My understanding as a young personal trainer in the 1990's was that in order to help people get in shape and live a healthful lifestyle I needed to know how they think, how they eat, and what demands they put on their bodies. I started my educational career on a premed track, graduating with a Bachelor of Science in athletic training, with minors in psychology, nutrition, and education. I was well on my way into the world of medicine when a severe injury during training changed my path. I went through the medical model of pain management, searching for a "cure" until meeting a sports chiropractor at a personal training forum who changed my life. During a presentation, he evaluated me from head to toe and without any knowledge of my history asked if I had been having mid-back pain.

Never having heard of a chiropractor at that moment, I was extremely intrigued because here was a man with no knowledge about me, yet understanding exactly my struggles with pain. He did not know my failed treatment history of receiving countless evaluations, x-rays, MRIs, nerve conduction studies, and spinal steroid injections. Even more disheartening, all of this treatment had come from specialists I one day wanted to be like. After he gave me some basic education on proper training and made me realize that the exercises I was doing were building muscles but were physically costly and counterproductive, he also showed me some basic mobilization movements that are now considered mainstream functional movement exercises; within two weeks of sticking to this routine, I found that my pain had subsided immensely. That relief did not just make me happy; it changed my mindset on the kind of doctor I wanted to be.

Throughout my chiropractic student career, I was lucky enough to have the opportunity to shadow many doctors, but one stood out from the pack, a sports chiropractor out of Brooklyn NY who had a huge patient base through the Public- School Athletic Leagues. Mostly he specialized in football and track and field injuries. It was not so much his amazing clinical or manual skills that I was impressed by but his humbling ability to not follow the latest gimmick or craze on the market. He strongly believed if patients are educated well and follow through with his guidance, most of their problems can be resolved. Jumping through the hoops of my chiropractic education required a singular belief tremendously preached in school: the body's innate ability to heal itself entirely through the alleviation of spinal segmental restrictions, also known as chiropractic subluxations. But my having had such an extensive background in human anatomy, physiology, emergency medical systems, and athletic training made me feel like an atheist sitting in church and listening to the gospels. Further, graduating from chiropractic school is like being born into the wild with no parental protection. You are strictly on your own and have to develop tough skin to handle everything that can possibly come in the door. Chiropractic graduates are not provided any system that can educate and promote their clinical excellence, such as a hospital system. Instead, many of us are compelled to open on our own and run a practice to the best of our ability by trial and error. All of my education throughout my career was in the mindset of getting my players back on their respective fields, with trial and error, until we got it right. I have strayed away from common mainstream beliefs that a patient needs to be under my care "Forever."

These beliefs have developed over the years with newfound research in the muscle skeletal world, which helps me express exactly what it is my manual skill sets allow me to do. Understanding that also makes me believe that since every person is so complexly unique, then there can't be a simple approach to their optimal health and well-being. When I first started my career as a chiropractor, I realized pretty quickly that manipulation was just a tool in my practitioner utility belt and not at all the means to a full resolve of symptoms. Patients would leave my office feeling better but always came back for more. If I were a salesman, it would be the perfect scenario to keep your customers coming back— but at what price?

As a holist, I believe I am what any healthcare practitioner ought to be: not a restricted specialist, but someone who has qualities of a humble empath, a practitioner who takes in everything and doesn't automatically reach conclusions or respond emotionally but instead takes time to know the client as an individual person. Soon, the humble empath develops a third eye, an experience-based sixth sense about each client. To arrive at health-promoting diagnoses, all health care practitioners must be non-judgmental, accepting clients' excuses bred and reinforced in their subconscious, and quietly listening to their rationalized or misinterpreted blaming. Soon, a game plan can be strategized for each individual and, as the client opens up, more will be accomplished appropriate to her or his needs. For me, being a good doctor means that the client must have an "aha" moment. The "aha" moment is when they realize what it truly takes to keep them at optimal health.

For many it becomes ritualized in daily routines that turn into habitual self- motivated processes through nutrition, movement, sleep, meditation, and mentally focused recovery. Nothing in life can be genuinely appreciated without work and determination. A person's health is a forever process which changes constantly, and the only way to conquer it is to stay ahead in the game of life.

Therapy, in my opinion, is a two-way street and cannot ever be attained solely by the practitioner. In no way do I take any responsibility away from the practitioner to be a good evaluator, educator, skilled provider, and coach. Detective work has become my therapeutic motive as a wellness practitioner; the questions I ask come from experience not just with what I have been trained to ask, but with investigation taken from these other modalities. The result is that frequently I must take a different, non-standard approach.

My first session starts with reciprocal education between myself and the patient or client. Even my introduction has been thought through over the years: now I walk into a room always smiling, because a serious look can be interpreted to be too serious and at times intimidating. As I enter a room, I tend to introduce myself as Dr. Vlad, my way of starting the relationship without making things too formal; rather than emphasizing a white coat and stethoscope, I accentuate a big smile, warm heart, and a personal name attached to the teddy bear exterior that is there for them, ready to listen observantly.

As the years have developed my education, I have changed many of my procedures, specifically when they come to evaluation. I no longer use only the standard approach of taking a simple history, performing a fundamental neurological and a focal orthopedic exam, and then beginning treatment. The history is always important, but many times does not express the actual reason they are in the office. To effectively assess their prognosis, I need to know their motives and how they think in order to stimulate them toward not only a successful outcome but a long-lasting one. Most of my cases I wish were as simple as a sprain or strain of one body part or region. However, a typical case may reveal not just a flare-up in one specific body part, but usually also in other regions found during the session that require attention but aren't as expressive as the primary region.

The fun begins when the patient presents herself with the problem, not knowing what could possibly have triggered her injury or pain in the first place. Where do we go if all we had was the basic questioning of what, where, when, and how? Unfortunately, most of what the patient can relay is usually too subjective, because opinions and recollections sometimes have emotional connections but are not facts. This kind of information is truly limited and can be used only in the background while objectively investigating. My objective examinations start with a theoretical construct developed by two heavy hitters in the fitness and physical therapy world, Gray Cook and Michael Boyle. Called the Joint-by-Joint approach, it represents a common association between each part of the body and its relation to the ones closest to it above and below. This theory, which focuses on alternating patterns of stability and mobility from one anatomical region to another, promotes the understanding that certain areas like your ankles, hips, shoulders, and thoracic need to express more mobility, while the feet, knees, lumbar (low back), and cervical spine (neck) need to appreciate stability. More specifically, mobility can be appreciated in a region when there is enough muscle extensibility to complete a statistically normal range of motion passively and actively under load; stability includes the timing and neuromuscular motor control of a region. Understanding this intricate balance between mobility and stability allows us to focus on things we need to help move and things we need to stabilize. Along with the Joint- by-Joint approach is the Selective Functional Movement Assessment, SFMA, a diagnostic system created to evaluate basic movement relationships with known musculoskeletal pain. It helps guide me to the most dysfunctional movement patterns that are not always expressive of pain but are usually a huge contributor to the pain-generating tissue.

Patients and I take the evaluation further for understanding what makes them tick by knowing about their habits, careers, and family interaction to translate what their average daily movement patterns and emotional well-being could be. After taking a history of what their current complaints are and prior injuries, we start with a selective functional movement assessment where we look at how they generally move, just like peeling the layers of an onion, homing in on their neuromuscular deficiencies and probable pain generators producing their symptoms. We progress from unloaded to loaded movement to begin to differentiate between structural limitations, functional limitations, or both. Palpatory skill sets are used to further define reflexively guarded muscle tissue that could be the primary cause of pain and dysfunction or dig further through the web of muscular layers, connecting junctions, and joint connections to find a secondary culprit of pain origin. Within the same palpatory process I also evaluate specific joint movement, taking note which joints lack movement and which might be overworking.

Once we have defined the patient's deficiencies, we begin the process physically, but the education starts immediately with the understanding that this will be a two-way street. You see, my job is to take the last few decades of clinically researched information, bottle it up into a digestible, easy to understand informative protocol for the client to absorb. The understanding has to be made that the biomechanical world of therapy has been constantly updating, with new theories of what is actually occurring in the body. Prior was a simpler understanding of just stretch and strengthening to recover from injury. With a newfound organ system such as the muscle skeletal fascial system and its vast sensory network, we have developed a better understanding of how our skin and fascia play a role affecting the body. Consequently, I have had to stay current with these newly developing theories and techniques, and frequently, although I understood them, I could not always fully explain them to a patient; maybe that was because each theory and technique wasn't actually a singular idea or process, its effects extensive and complicated.

As time proceeded, I began to learn that combinations of therapies yielded even more effective results. In my office I feel as if I'm the composer of a synchronous variety of modalities to produce my melody of manual input for the patient's brain to be subdued for a better appreciation of pain information. During a typical treatment session, the patient's body and mind are being stimulated with different modalities. We start with a relaxing process with heat (diathermy) to increase blood flow and increase muscle relaxation, and electric muscle stimulation to decrease muscle tone, increase circulation, and desensitize the targeted areas. Once the body is relaxed, I use not only topical creams to decrease friction on the skin, but also penetrating compounds such as capsaicin, menthol, and/or CBD to affect pain receptors by desensitizing them. I apply soft and/or deep tissue massage to continue mobilizing the tissue to promote fluid distribution, increase blood flow, and decrease muscle tone. I introduce Instrument Assisted Soft Tissue Mobilization (IASTM) to the prepped tissue to facilitate the healing process through increased fibroblast proliferation and increased collagen synthesis, maturation, and alignment to break up myofascial adhesions. To further promote tissue glide and reperfusion, I might incorporate some soft tissue flossing. After the use of all of these compressive forces I will decompress the tissue with cupping therapy, further promoting increased blood flow and decreasing pain sensitization. Once the soft tissue has been released, relaxed, and vascularized, I now have a window of opportunity to properly affect the joints that are restricted and lack movement with the use of various Joint Mobilizations and Grade 5 Manipulations (AKA Chiropractic Adjustment or Osteopathic Manipulation). Joint mobilization and manipulation promote better movement with stimulation of mechanoreceptors, reflexively relaxing muscle tissue, and breaking up fibrous adhesions within the joint, allowing it to move properly.

Once the patient and I have convinced the body to relax, I continue by instilling movement through static and dynamic flexibility to increase range of motion and promote, in a sense, a muscle memory to the new range the muscles have expressed. Typically depending on the patient's skin sensitivity, an application of kinesiology taping will be applied to promote continual therapy for a few more days by consistently feeding the skin with information to actively inhibit pain through sensory mechanoreceptor activation. All of these stimulations, when the patient leaves, carry with them a spillover effect for the next few days. Keep in mind that my practice is principally designed, or specified, to be physical, and in this exact moment is actually where the magic happens.

Once patients have experienced some relief or in many cases an unloading of stress, they begin to accept some of my future suggestions and next steps. What I have realized is that my treatment sessions are important but are most definitely not the sum of patients' whole recovery. My therapy is only a gateway for continued self- care. My clients develop a better understanding that body work is one piece and that the other pieces have to come together with how they think, what they put into their bodies, and how they move.

My professional and personal experience with doctors has taught me that wellness will be insufficient if a doctor does not have a network of contacts. Keeping my ego always checked, I understand that I too have limitations out of my eclectically informed specialty. This is also because every individual is a complex, many-pieced puzzle that often requires additional experts either to see the whole therapeutic picture, or to bring in new pieces to make that puzzle more complete and more visible, thus more holistic. I rely on a set of colleagues related to my patients' needs. These needs definitely have therapeutic layers guiding whom to refer to. First, we put out the fire when a specialization is needed for a focal and specialized approach such as orthopedics, neurology, anesthesiology, etc. But when the fire is out, we must find the reason for the fire so it doesn't happen again. The chronic or insidious reasons require a biopsychosocial intervention, and therefore solution to clients' needs will range from a functional medicine practitioner and/or nutritional consultation to subdue their inflammatory markers, to a psychological consult to address biopsychosocial limitations, and/or a personal training life coach to solidify the movements we achieved in our therapy session for improved performance. This accessibility of colleagues allows patients to have accountability to achieve their goals.

Their part starts with the understanding that their body's healing has its own process, its own timeframe, its own reality. They must begin to be more mindful of what their body is telling them—and no, igno-rance is not bliss. Having a high pain threshold is no longer sexy when you try to accomplish optimal health. Pain is your best expressive sen-sory motivation to help you change the demand you are unknowingly placing on your body. After all the physicality that I perform within a session and the client leaves the office, with improvement, is when the true healing process actually begins.

Therapy and the body's ability to adapt and heal is the process. A misconception brought to my office, often, is that my treatment will be like a "Hollywood Chiropractic" scene. The patient will be placed on the table, and I will "Presto Chango!" their body with a forever pain-free life. Now that would be an amazing superpower, but unfortunately that is not how true therapy works. Fortunately, instead of superpowers we have prior and current wisdoms that have been passed on from a multitude of practitioners and researchers to help us guide what we can do. Many times, the hardest part is remembering to do them all. There-fore, it is truly not a commitment to me that I require of patients but a holistically multivariable commitment to themselves. This dedication is not an overnight success, as this commitment comes usually within the process and it is my job to help my clients reach an "Ah-ha" mo-ment, when recognition comes to them and they get results they have not seen before, driven by needs that are not necessarily performed by the specialist. Any application performed on the body passively or ac-tively has a multivariable dosage-to-recovery response time. For exam-ple, performing soft tissue mobilization on a 6-foot, 220 pound, 25 year-old professional athlete will be totally different from working on a 5'6", 140 pound, 55 year-old working woman with comorbidities. How you recover is many times directly proportionate to what kind of environment you provide for your body. If the body is young, oxygenated, and nutrient dense, the probability of a faster recovery is certain. If the body is, in a sense, fighting within itself, the recovery time takes longer. This is why patients need to affirm a true commitment to themselves in order to provide a proper environment for healing and recovery.

Everything that I have mentioned seems to boil down to one concept: any person, when considered a complex puzzle requiring the integration of so many possible pieces, will be better managed by professional advisors than by doing it alone. The patients that have had the most productive success in their outcomes have all had realizations that their approach must be a multivariable approach just as their lives have a multivariable road. One patient comes to mind who has had what I would call an extraordinary life and has become a gracious student of his own body. Genetically he wasn't dealt such a great hand of cards, as he has had a slew of problems that came on throughout his life, none relating back to his lifestyle. With persistence of seeking out guidance from many professionals with different backgrounds, he now has the luxury of not only appreciating life but actually still having one. This is a man in his seventies who has checked his ego with his body a long time ago. He has many people he holds close to keep him biopsychosocially accountable, starting close to home with his amazing wife, and bolstered by the three professionals he sees weekly: his lifestyle performance coach, a fitness trainer of over 18 years who keeps him in check nutritionally and challenges his heart, breath, and body in general; his Pilates coach, who keeps his mind connected to his body under strenuous demands; and his manual therapist, who helps his body recover from the demands he puts on his body weekly. When things arise unexpectedly or when he decides on a new goal to achieve that might be out of the scope of practice or knowledge from his immediate advisors, he will reach into his rolodex to access his team of other practitioners for guidance, a cardiologist for his bypassed heart, a urologist for his prostate cancer, an endocrinologist for his diabetes, a podiatrist for his slightly neuropathic feet, an ophthalmologist for his blind right eye, an ear specialist for his deaf left ear. This is a man who had his "aha" moment a long time ago and now continues to appreciate his journey. That's what this book is about: a collection of health care providers from different fields helping you understand how to appreciate your physical and mental lifestyle journey.

As you will see, "what can I do or where should I start?" is sometimes a very hard question to answer. Fortunately, I've asked a few of my colleagues to help me answer these questions and much more through their own personal and professional perspective to help you define what you should do and where you could start. Our aim is for you to be able to understand the different components of health and optimal living and to help you begin your journey of creating a mindful game plan for an optimal life. Throughout this book we will help you better understand the biopsychosocial fundamentals and where to begin, with behavior modification and habit change strategies to help you implement the process of change. For you to build confidence to overcome pain, a true understanding of physical and emotional pain is a must to build a resilient body and mind. Throughout my years in practice I've realized that what you put into your body directly relates to how it and your mind will function—the ability to understand that there truly is a difference between living to eat and eating to live. That is why we have included a plethora of information on fundamental nutrition and diseases that easily develop from our Standard American Diet. We hope to enlighten you on how to be aware of your dietary individuality and point you in a better direction of customizing your nutrition and lifestyle based on your health concerns. Regeneration and recovery are the buzz-words mostly used in the health and fitness industry, and understanding the fundamental biopsychosocial necessities of nutrition, sleep, and stress management will guide you to better recovery from physical and mental stress. It has been known for the last few decades that the Western world has accepted many philosophies and techniques from the Eastern world, so as holists we introduce some Eastern medicine practices and protocols for authentic living. Movement, in my opinion, is the key to your body's life; as I mention to my patients, the only time you don't need to move is when you are six feet under. Yes, as grim as that sounds, it's still the truth. If you're not moving, you're dying. It can be seen very simply once an individual is casted for a broken limb. To promote bone healing, we at times must restrict movement of the affected limb and, once the cast is taken off (usually 6-8 weeks), muscle atrophy is immediately appreciated. Therefore, movement is truly one of the most important facets for optimal health, and in this book we bring you the most common practices known from the worlds of yoga, Pilates, and strength training. When your mind conceives and perceives what needs to be done, your body will achieve it. But dreams without goals are just wishes, which is why we have also included some information for SMART goal setting, to understand personal baselines and how to progress your routines with a focus on movement and training applications.

CHAPTER II

Biopsychosocial Fundamentals of Wellness

Hicham Haouzi

I've always had an interest in sports, and my athletic background includes playing soccer first, then learning and competing in Taekwondo, kickboxing, and Muay Thai. Member of the Moroccan 1988 Olympics Taekwando team, I studied Muay Thai in Thailand between 1992-1995, during which time I won the 1992-3 Dutch Muay Thai boxing competition. Moving to the U.S., I then won the U.S. 1999 Excaliber Muay Thai Challenge gold medal and, later, another gold medal at the first U.S. national Muay Thai competition in 2001, which placed me on the national team. Beginning as an Equinox trainer in 2000, I attained the fitness company's highest ranking trainer position, Tier-X, in 2004. Since then I've received the Equinox Lifetime Achievement award in 2012, co-founded and become a member of the Equinox Olympic Committee, which for three consecutive years promoted Equinox Games, and now am General Manager of Hudson Yards' E Training Studios in Manhattan, the most elite coaching platform offered by Equinox. Additionally, I have worked at Mt. Sinai Hospital's Rehab Center for Addiction, training one-on-one with patients to promote their physical movement, coached soccer teams, individual celebrities and high-profile business people, and have certifications including the 21-credit NYU Program in Business and Coaching.

I mention my history as a competitive athlete and fitness trainer because my credentials show how much time I spent learning and experiencing new theories, techniques, and challenges about health, wellness, and longevity, and in particular the fundamental practices needed to live properly. These fundamental abilities not only have helped me to continue to improve my daily tasks, but will help me to share with you all that's needed for biopsychosocial wellness, managing properly and efficiently the body, mind, and surrounding influences in life. Wellness requires multitasking, a fluid integration of reactions to accomplish a goal without negatively affecting our objective. This biopsychosocial multitasking cannot be properly achieved without first knowing the fundamentals introduced and explained in this chapter. Everything in life has a base, a proper way of how to start it, a foundation upon which to build it. Therefore, if you lack foundations or fundamentals, the primary rules or principles, you will not succeed fully or solidly or last longer efficiently throughout the process of your life. Any changes from learning and mastering all of these biopsychosocial fundaments will come when each of you has the courage to question your own fundamental values and beliefs and then see to it that your actions lead to your best intentions.

I. The Mind

A. Mental conditioning

No matter what you are setting out to accomplish, the very first step to getting you to where you want to go begins with the mind. Your thinking has so much power over your ability to reach your goals, and it's very important to recognize that your thoughts, attitudes, and beliefs are both choices and skills. This is good news because just like any other skills, these can be learned and improved with practice. Mental conditioning is a process of training your mind to modify your thoughts, attitudes, and beliefs to accept thinking patterns, tendencies, and/or mental states in order to optimize positive thinking and ultimately optimize your performance. When you become aware of your thinking patterns and assess your starting point, it's from this baseline that you can intentionally set a path forward to practice in areas where you'd like to see improvements that will translate into both increased performance and quality of life.

This is true for each of the fundamentals of the mind that follow below. By focusing in these areas, you will build a strong foundation of practice in using your thinking as a powerful tool to create the mental meaning, focus, flexibility, and stamina that we all need in the journey towards our goals. At the core of each of these is practicing to keep your mindset to stay in the present moment. In other words, keeping an emphasis on only the now and returning to it again and again when you find yourself drifting away from the moment. This helps to prohibit stress and anything else destructive that we might bring to an exercise session.

B. Positivity-motivation (Positivity feeds motivation.)

A positive state of mind is one that continues to seek, find, and execute ways to win or to find a desirable outcome, regardless of the circumstances. This concept is the opposite of negativity, defeatism, and hopelessness. It is living by the philosophy of finding greater joy in small joys and to live without hesitation or holding back our most cherished personal virtues and values. Optimism and hope are vital to developing and nurturing a positive mindset that will help you to sustain the motivation and problem-solving skills needed to carry you through mastering new skills, inevitable challenges, and unpredicted set-backs.

C. Openness for mental clarity = Understanding

Communication and education are the building blocks both to understanding and to a strong relationship that is based on trust. Why is this important? Because you can't trust something that you don't understand. What are you personally doing and why? What is the process and the science behind your plan? These questions should be part of ongoing conversations between the coach and the client because, without experience, the client will not necessarily know why they are doing something. I like to ask my clients this question, "Would you rather be the sail boat or the wind?" I like it because it is a good solid question to make them stop for a second and become aware of both their thought process and where they stand. It helps to clear up their identity a bit by bringing awareness to what drives them and what they want. Sometimes, who they think they are is not actually who they really are. and what they think they want is not actually what they really want. There is no right or wrong answer—just useful insight into their mind in that moment and an opportunity to consider, "Is that really what I want? Is it working for me?" Keeping an openness to taking a closer look at the why behind what drives you and all the elements of your plan is the path to greater mental clarity and understanding. This helps to build trust in your coach, in your plan, and within yourself.

D. Acceptance of capability

Acceptance of capability is about setting realistic goals, motivation, and injury prevention. If you can accept your capabilities in the present moment, then you also are setting yourself up for feeling encouraged, building motivation, and preventing injuries that could set you back in your plan. So what are you capable of today? How does this match with your stated goals? It is here that coaching becomes critical. Some coaches, in an effort to keep the client happy, just stay on plan. But the best coaches know that creating an exercise program and successfully executing it requires constant attention to your current capabilities and builds into it the flexibility to adjust your incremental goals to meet you where you are today, in the present moment. Here are just a few examples of when the conversation with your coach needs to come back to the present moment to discuss your current capabilities, what could go wrong (injury), and include a path forward toward the goal that also matches your current capabilities.

1. You come into an exercise session stating as a physical goal that you want to do 10 pull-ups, but the reality is that you don't yet have the conditioning to achieve this goal safely and would be better served with an incremental plan to build up to 10 pull-ups.

2. You've been up all night with your kids and you come to the gym on 2 hours of sleep and tell your coach that you "want to crush it today," but a lighter workout would allow you to still condition and not further exhaust your body when it really needs recovery.

3. You have the mental goal of wanting to squat 150 lbs., but you need understanding to accept that you are physically not able to squat 150 lbs. and that attempting something not meant for your body is not good for your health and well-being.

It is human nature to want to push limits, but you have to be able to say to yourself, "It's OK. I can accept the reality of where I am and will pull back for the moment so that I am able to move forward and keep progressing on the larger plan." Sometimes it is hard to accept these limitations. This is especially true for over-achievers and for people who are aging. When you approach 40-50 years of age, it can be really challenging to learn what your new limitations are. It's like walking a tight rope between your mind and body of what you used to be able to do, what you now can do, what you shouldn't do, and alternatives. Here, coaching becomes so much more important, as the focus needs to shift to injury prevention and longevity and not to continue bench pressing as much as possible and going to the beach. That's how you know that you are in good hands: when the coach helps you to take a step back in order for you to be able to continue to move forward to prevent new injuries and limitations so you can continue on your path toward your goals. A huge part of this relationship is trust. Trust has to come from the beginning. It is rooted in transparency of the plan and expectations, and then it takes a little time for actions and situations to build up as proof you can trust that person. You shouldn't expect to have trust in day one. Both coach and client have to show commitment and actions that demonstrate to each other that they can trust each other.

When you accept your current capabilities and have established trust with your coach, you will be receptive to his or her communication and recommendations—but make no mistake, you still own your decisions. For example, if you are training hard and your coach recommends that you pull back a bit and take the weekend off for recovery, it is a suggestion. Your coach cannot decide for you. It is still you who needs to decide that you will take the weekend off so that you can feel that much better on Monday; on Monday, when you perform better, that's ownership.

E. Expectations/Commitment

Commitment is the state of being dedicated to a cause or activity. It is tied to ownership, but it's not the same. Commitment is tangible. For example, I can ask you, on a level from 1-10, how committed are you to your fitness program? If you answer 8, my next questions are going to be a) Why are you an 8 and not a 10? and b) How can we make it a 10? If you tell me that it's because you can only work out twice per week, this is tangible and now we have a starting point for more discussion. You can't reinforce the commitment of someone if they are not committed. It's up to them. It's also useful to mention that if someone can commit to an 8, the actual output more likely will be between a 6 and an 8 because of the inevitable things in life that can pull you back at times (people get sick, injured, etc.).

It's good to be aware of this and to set expectations that not everything is going to go the way you planned. Communication between client and coach along these lines should be honest. The coach cannot simply tell the client what they want to hear, but rather the coach has to tell the client what they think is right for them in that moment. It's very important here to use the proper language with the client so they understand. This language has to be tailored, meaning all clients cannot be treated the same. You need to know how to speak to each client individually, based on the language they understand, the relationship, level of trust, knowledge, and their experience. It has to be simple, clear, honest, direct, and short—not a speech. This is a skill the coaches have to work on themselves to have the confidence and trust in themselves to know who can be pushed and who cannot—not because they can't be pushed, but because it won't work. Certainly here, experience can help.

F. Ownership

Self-ownership means being comfortable in your own shoes and owning your attitudes and actions. People with self-ownership take responsibility for their lives. They have exceptional self-confidence, which allows them to unconditionally love themselves and accept their minor imperfections. So how do you trigger self-confidence and foster ownership? A good starting point is for the client to answer the critical question of "Why are they there?" and "What is their goal and the reasons behind it?" I ask these questions because it's hard to reinforce confidence if there's no clarity around the goal. During this discussion, as a coach, I take myself out of the equation. The coach should not set the goal because, if the coach sets the goal, this kills ownership on day one, leaving nothing that the client can own after that. Now, the coach is in charge. So this is important: the client must set the goal. Here are some examples of how this could take shape and some strategies to address them:

1. They have a clear goal and know why they want it, but they are not confident. A strategy here could be to look to draw upon other parts of their life in which they are or were very confident so they can tap into what it feels like and be able to envision it in this new space

2. They have a clear goal, but the goal isn't realistic. For example, someone who has never run before stating that they want to run a marathon within 6 months. This situation calls for the coach to be honest, but not discouraging, by providing a gentle reality check and laying out a plan that starts with building a base and then building upon that base in phases towards incremental goals.

3. They don't really know what they are there for, or they are just there because they see someone else doing it (social media, celebrity, friend). This situation requires more discussion and search for mental clarity, which can take time over several discussions, so it's good to approach this with patience.

With all these scenarios you can draw upon these answers to give guidance and set up the client for success by assessing their starting point and making a plan with realistic outcomes and expectations that also creates opportunities for incremental wins which build their self-confidence along the way.

Seeing the starting point of where you are and having clarity on where you want to go, along with clear steps to take to get there, is a journey to self- ownership. When you decide what you want from deep inside of you, and you work hard through obstacles to achieve what you believe you want, you own it. No one can take it away from you. And that in itself is very powerful in fitness and in life.

G. Motivation: When you have ownership, that gives you motivation.

Motivation, derived from the word motive or a need that requires satisfaction, is a reason for actions, willingness, and goals. These needs, wants, or desires may be acquired either through the influence of culture, society, and lifestyle (outside forces, which are extrinsic motivations), or may be generally innate (intrinsic motivations). Considered one of the most important reasons to move forward, motivation results from the interaction of both conscious and unconscious factors. Mastering motivation to allow sustained and deliberate practice is central to high levels of achievement, in elite sports, medicine, music, or any practiced skill. Motivation governs choices among alternative forms of voluntary activity.

For sustainable motivation, one should tap into the motivation coming from a meaningful place inside of you, to understand what drives your need. This involves reflecting on what drives you to want what you want. This is found in the moments that you sit deep with yourself and try to connect to the inside instead of outside—not the exterior drivers, but what drives you to do something inside, that really connects you with yourself. That is the true motivation. That's what will really get you to complete a task or a goal without creating obstacles or dropping the tasks that will get you there. For example, if you want to run because your neighbors are running, but you hate running and yet I give you a program for running, what is going to happen in 3 weeks? With the passage of time, it will become increasingly challenging to sustain the extrinsic motivation to keep training. It's easier to simply lose the drive to continue at the first sight of challenge.

In contrast, if you want to run because of a need or desire that you are deeply connected with, you are more likely to sustain your motivation to push through challenges and towards your goal. If your desire to run is meaningful to you so that, for example, you are fit and capable to run behind your child while they learn to ride a bicycle, this is a connected meaning that is much more likely to sustain your intrinsic motivation through the inevitable challenges ahead.

Deep meaning will sustain your drive. Everyone has this inside motivation; some people are aware of it and some people have to work hard to discover it.

H. Meditation

Whereas the preceding paragraphs about mental fundamentals follow a sequence of preparation, the practice of meditation can occur any time throughout your mental preparedness. Meditation trains you to give oxygen to the mind and body and to calm your biopsycho operations. The distribution of oxygen to the body helps to settle down the mind's energy and to prepare for the upcoming physical task, by again reminding a person to enter the present, the now.

Meditation helps you to discover how you feel emotionally and where in your body any tension or irregularity is felt (e.g. neck, lower back). Then, wherever stress is most intense, put yourself in a relaxing position to take stress off that area; in this position there will be no gravity. Placing the back of your head on the floor and your body in a supine position, with knees bent, will change the entire dynamic of how you feel; this is what on a very basic level yoga attempts to accomplish, helping you to find balance and to remove stress. Furthermore, beyond breathing, visualizations and sounds can be added to attain meditative benefits. Visual imaging, which can increase psychological peace, helps anyone to feel better about the past and to prepare for the future: by seeing a joyful image, such as crossing the finish line of an upcoming race or being a future grandparent playing actively with grandchildren, we can set an optimistic tone in our psyche. Hearing actual tones or sound from music, a mantra, or from any external vibration, or even silence, goes through your body to promote circulation and energy flow in an attempt to synchronize with human brain waves to de-stress the body. This purity attained through visual and tonal receptivity is accomplished partially by allowing thoughts to come and go without consciously processing or directing them. In effect, relaxed breathing with visualization and sound will help the meditator to pacify the soul.

II. The Body

A. Breathing

If you don't breathe properly, your body won't function properly, because it needs to be fed with oxygen. The only thing that doesn't change throughout your life, from your birth to your death, breathing is a fundamental part of your existence; you can't have circulation, or life, without breathing first. The first thing to become irregular when people are stressed or feel any kind of emotion is their breath.

1.   Breathing at Rest: Lying on your back with your knee bent, breathe through the nose, not through the mouth. Keep your shoulders relaxed, and place your hands on the belly. Take a couple of minutes to relax.

2.   After a couple of minutes, ask yourself where you are feeling tension: in the belly, chest, shoulders, neck? Creating awareness of where tension is felt, with gravity taken out of the equation, you will realize the source of why you're not breathing diaphragmatically. The diaphragm opens your lungs for performance and recovery. Now, take a deep breath through your nose with hands still on the belly, and feel your belly filling with air like a balloon. As a guiding inhale/exhale ratio with this breathing, inhale for one and exhale for three. When you exhale, the opposite of the inhale should happen: the balloon deflates. This basic ratio will change when the body performs different techniques, as in yoga or when exercising.

53

B. Set your goals for success.

What is a "smart goal"? A smart goal:

1. must have specific metrics, be measurable, for example a distance (run one mile?), a length in time (a one-mile run under nine minutes?), a number of pounds and repetitions (ten biceps curls with 30 pounds?)

2. is attainable or achievable. Can you realistically accomplish this goal, and do you have the skill needed?

3. is guided by a time frame: have you set a date for when you want to achieve this goal? Because you will start modestly, will that allow you enough time to achieve it?

4. is informed by relevance and realism:
   a) is the goal worthwhile?
   b) is this the right time to achieve this goal?
   c) are you honest with yourself that you're capable both mentally and physically to achieve this goal?
   d) test yourself first to know if the goal is realistic, and be certain that you're prepared to work within the deadline you've set.

C. Set-up and needed tools

Set-up refers to your biopsychosocial preparedness for your bodily goals, which includes all factors to guarantee your workout's success: proper sleep and nutrition; hydration before and water during the workout; guaranteed privacy or separation, without needless interruptions from environmental demands of work, family, and other external responsibilities. Have at hand whatever equipment you will need, such as mat, weights, bars.

D. Acceptance of challenges, where synergy must enter

Self-awareness of capabilities is essential. You must be able to accept your limitations and challenges. If needed, look for easier versions and readjust your goals. Focus on what you can do, not on what you can't. Remember that you are competing against yourself, not against others. Keep in mind your goals for success.

E. Practice/practice/practice;

With A through D formulated, you now are prepared to teach your body to achieve success with your goals. Improvement of all skills requires practice, whether it's playing piano, writing essays, or shooting or dribbling a basketball. With practice you develop your skill sets.

F. Self-reward

Throughout the process of attaining your goals, be sure to acknowledge your accomplishments and to pat yourself on the back. From a successful workout comes an elevated mood, so congratulate yourself that you are one step closer to your goals. Self-reward includes giving yourself a break from your routine: take off the weekend, enjoy a good walk, see a movie, get a massage. Literally bring the synergy of your biopsycho accomplishment to the social context, so that your feeling of wellness becomes biopsychosocial. Total ownership of the product your process has led to is the purpose of setting goals. With that comes a sense of completion and fulfillment.

III. Synergy

We can refer to the blending or merging of energy between the mind and the body as synergy; it's an interaction that becomes a unity or union, a harmony or alliance. In effect, synergy is an efficiency resulting from trial and error which leads to a coordinated balance of expended energy while still being in the moment and able to adapt to different needs.

One of the goals of synergy is energy efficiency, which simply means using less energy to perform the same task – that is, eliminating energy waste. Energy efficiency brings a variety of benefits: reducing greenhouse gas emissions, reducing demand for energy imports, and lowering our costs on a household and economy-wide level. On a personal level, energy efficiency also can be attained, through a person's developed implementation of synergy.

A useful analysis of synergic blending within my mind and body occurred when at 51 years-old I competed in the 2020 New York City Marathon. My mental and bodily training of course included all the fundamentals discussed here. Because synergy is a developmental process, its product during the marathon was how well I handled the marathon competitively. It's important to know that I had trained to compete not against other runners but against a time-goal I'd set: below four hours. My motivation therefore was a personal goal, and my preparatory fundamentals were conditioned by that.

Despite whatever goals or necessities you may have trained for, the competitive moment requires a dialogue between your mind and body from beginning to end, a synergy changing itself as changes occur. Two times while running the marathon I was challenged by a bodily/mental imbalance or lack of coordination. First was when, between miles 18 and 20, I became physically challenged due to the dead silence on the bridge from the Bronx to Manhattan, a span with no people, no distractions, and a lack of external energy literally encouraging me, only the sound of feet pounding; that was when mental energy needed to become a restorative influence. As I felt my body slowing, legs heavier, with awareness of my breathing, questions at that moment began to fill my mind about my body's abilities, and I wondered if I should quit or maybe just slow down. Then, my synergic training brought focus into the moment, setting one coordinated mental/physical goal: to get off the bridge and out of that area. And suddenly the focus on my lethargic legs and butt was removed, refocusing instead to look for the next crowd to provide me with further energy. Back to life again and aware that I was 3/4 done with the race and back in Manhattan with crowds, I knew I was going to make it. And, with that, I returned to a focus on my finishing time.

Another moment of challenge came at mile 22, when I couldn't get my body to accelerate. So, I dialogued with myself, forgot about my body, shifted the focus away from speed, and started looking at people, using them as a series of targets to reach, one person after another, until the finish line. Unlike many people who "hit the wall" and stop at this point in the race—four miles to go—I was able to shift mentally, make a quick decision in the moment, and set a new goal that was attainable.

Running the NY City Marathon was an amazing learning experience! Not only about running, it also was about what you have in your core. You have run—depleted— all the strength, all the superficial fitness out of yourself, and it really comes down to what's left inside you. The POWER OF THE MIND! To be able by using my synergy to draw deep and pull something out of myself is one of the most tremendous things that I feel today about my experience running the NY City Marathon!

IV. Spiritual and Emotional = Social

When working to attain biopsychosocial wellness, there's a third fundamental that's additional to preparedness of the body(bio) and the mind (psycho): spiritual and emotional aspects of our being (social).

The Spirit fundamental

Like the word wellness, spirit is fraught with multiple meanings. Wherever the sources of its meanings stem from—religion, philosophy, psychology, physics, neuroscience—we know that spirit seeks purpose and in our own life and in how we live it. Our spirit must partner wisely with peaceful acceptance and respect for what exists beyond our self: family, trusted friends, and the duties required by them: unconditional love, guidance, and support, whether through religious instruction or through ethical codes of behavior. Supporting one's family is attained through a person's or a couple's work, and through professional income, which can create stress. Further stress can arise from inescapable social and cultural realities surrounding us, especially those found in broadcast media and in printed news, which reproduce politics and economics and add to our stress.

How we receive, interpret, and manage natural and manmade forces depends on our spirit. To know our spirit requires not only inspecting our world view, our values, and goals, but also peacefully learning to modify or eliminate our needless intolerances. Important to spiritual wellness is feeling true to oneself while being gentle with all that is not oneself.

The Emotional fundamental

All humans have feelings and emote. Awareness and acceptance of one's feelings is the first step toward emotional wellness; with that, we learn to see realistically our emotional limitations, emotionally charged behaviors, and emotional memories. This learning provides insights into how to manage our feelings and their related behaviors, and ultimately how to take responsibility for our actions. Through our self-awareness, we develop our ability to cope, to be self-reliant, and to generate positivity and enthusiasm about self and life. We face challenges, take risks, and recognize conflict as potentially advantageous. All of this leads to maintaining satisfying relationships with other people and to establishing social commitment, trust, and respect.

Emotional wellness helps us to live and work productively and to realize the importance of seeking and valuing the support and assistance of others. We are more likely to see life as an exciting, hopeful adventure, not as a fearful, bothersome, anxiety-producing struggle when our emotional being is in balance.

Possibly you've noticed while reading this chapter that so many of the different biopsychosocial fundamentals I've discussed interconnect and overlap with one another, creating new synergies which, if properly balanced, can respond to new demands and serve our immediate needs. This is natural, because we humans are multifaceted beings, complicated organisms whose functioning is itself interconnected and overlapping. With the fundamentals introduced and explained in this chapter, I've shared with you all that's needed to start on your path to biopsychosocial wellness, managing properly and efficiently the body, mind, and surrounding influences in life. In sum, it all can be boiled down to these three key elements of biopsychosocial health:

1. Mental conditioning, the process of training your mind to modify your thoughts, attitudes, and beliefs to accept new thinking patterns, tendencies, and/or mental states in order

to optimize positive thinking and ultimately optimize your performance.

2.   The body, a complex mechanism and organism, needs multiple factors to interact among each other for us to complete a task or a goal; this includes breathing, exercising, sleep, nutrition, hydration, and a synergistic relationship between the energies of the body and mind.

3.   Spiritual wellness, from which we derive meaning and purpose, is a feeling of being true to oneself while being gentle with all that is not oneself.

As you journey through the remaining chapters of this book, my colleagues will talk more and in greater detail about the aspects or theories that interact in the different ways I've described. It all falls under this master umbrella of biopsychosocial wellness. I wish for you that this chapter has given you some understanding and clarity of how we human beings function and that it brings you an awareness and knowledge about yourself—about the fundamentals of your mind, body, and spirit, which make up your biopsychosocial health as you seek to approach longevity and a better quality of life.

CHAPTER III

Changing Bad Habits for Good
Dr. Bob Davis and David Jean-Bart

Along with knowing the fundamentals of biopsychosocial wellness before dedicating yourself to a more healthful life, you should know conceptually and strategically how to break bad habits and, with behavior modification, to create good ones. Within psychology, "habitual behaviors are defined as actions triggered automatically when people encounter situations in which they have consistently done them in the past. Repeating behavior in the same context reinforces mental associations between the context and behavior." Prompted by environmental settings and their specific stimuli, we become conditioned to respond in habitual ways:

> Habit is said to have formed when exposure to the context nonconsciously activates the association, which in turn elicits an urge to act, influencing behavior with minimal conscious forethought. As an initially goal-directed behavior becomes habitual, control over behavior is transferred from a reasoned, reflective processing system, which elicits behavior relatively slowly based on conscious motivation, to an impulsive system, which elicits behavior rapidly and efficiently, based on learned context-behavior associations. Habitual behaviors thus become detached froconscious motivational processes (Gardner, 1).

Habitual behaviors detached from conscious motivational processes aren't necessarily detrimental or negative; in numerous contexts all of us have created and can continue to create conditioned behaviors benefiting our own and other people's life through positive reinforcement that becomes instinctual. The focus here, however, is to help you change whatever negative behaviors you have that may prohibit or be injurious to your biopsychosocial wellness. Behavior modification and habit change mean, first, that obviously you've concluded there's some compulsion or urge, pattern or practice in your life you need to change for some reason, whether it's to do whatever your doctors advise you to do, to make your partner and kids happier, or to make yourself satisfied and peaceful about who, what, and where you are physically, psychologically, socially, and economically.

Bad habits and limiting behaviors can be caused by innate human defiance, the need for social acceptance, the inability to truly understand the nature of risk, an individualistic view of the world and consequent rationalization of unhealthful habits, and a genetic predisposition to addiction (Bryner). Buried into your behavior, these causes of bad habits are triggered or cued principally either by stress or by boredom, but sources of stress and boredom are broadly various as influences, and the bad habits caused by them can be diverse. Willpower certainly will aid your determination to break bad habits, but there's no need to rely on it exclusively, just as there's no need to feel shame because of bad habits.

The first necessity for breaking bad habits and changing to beneficial new ones is to realize that everyone in the world, different by nature and nurture, has bad habits and behaviors warranting improvement or change; therefore, because nobody's perfect, you aren't alone if you want to make changes to improve. Possibly, the difficulty to make changes has increased because we live in an increasingly non-contemplative age of immediate gratification in which many people have very high and unrealistic expectations of theories and practices about habit change and consequently aren't willing to take the time to learn more about them and to test them. In some cases, many of us don't even truly understand what our own desired outcome should be for behavioral change and eliminating bad habits.

Breaking bad habits and changing to beneficial new ones also requires a second necessity, that you accept medical science's repeatedly proven finding observed here by Dr. Mark Hyman: your zip code is more of a determining factor of your health than your genetic code. "The story of your health is much more complex than genetic programming," Hyman writes. "It is ultimately determined by the dynamic interplay of the environment washing over genes creating the 'you' of this moment." Many of us have assumed that inheriting strong, favorable genetics allows us to get away with or withstand bad habits and behaviors which, although potentially injurious in other people, aren't likely to affect us negatively. Bury and forget that belief! Hyman informs us that the October 2010 issue of *Science* magazine "published an important paper that reviewed the notion of the 'exposome'—the idea that the environment in which your genes live is more important than your genes themselves. What this suggests is that applying genomics to treat disease is misguided because 70-90 percent of your disease risk is related to your environment exposures and the resultant alterations in molecules that wash over your genes" (Hyman). Please read that last sentence again, as it's an underlying presupposition helping to convince you of the importance of habit change. Exposomes come from what we eat, what we're conditioned to think, how we feel, environmental toxins, the microbiome (the collective genomes of the microbes—composed of bacteria, bacteriophage, fungi, protozoa, and viruses—that live inside and on the human body), our stress levels, poor nutrition, and a lack of exercise and sleep. Bathed daily in these exposomes, your genome is the recipient of a host of unhealthful, even harmful influences—if you allow it to be.

Obviously implied by this scientific reality is that you, yourself, can alter "the resultant alterations in molecules that wash over [your] genes" by changing your behaviors and habits, especially those that are damaging or "bad." Unlike the warning which you're given on a pack of cigarettes, far too many exposomes negatively impacting our lives don't offer warnings or even a hint of their detrimental influences. On many levels, therefore, behavior modification and habit change require additional awareness and new recognitions which you must discover and own. In this chapter we'll give insights guiding you to help yourself understand the values and priorities underlying your behavior; those insights will enable you to create a strategic approach to setting proper behaviors and habits that allow you to reap the benefits of living a full, biopsychosocially healthful life.

One of our favorite scientific processes with which to modify bad behavioral habits and to change to good ones is The Transtheoretical Model (TTM) or Stages of Change Model. Proposed in the late 1970s, TTM was developed through studies examining differences between the experiences of smokers who quit on their own and those of smokers requiring further treatment. These studies determined that people quit smoking only if they were ready to do so. Thus, TTM focuses on the decision-making of the individual and is a model of intentional change, operating on the assumption that people do not change behaviors quickly and decisively. Rather, change in behavior, especially habitual behavior, occurs continually through a cyclical process. Because "The TTM is not a theory but a model," we should remember that "different behavioral theories and constructs can be applied to various stages of the model where they may be most effective" (The Transtheoretical Model).

The TTM posits that individuals move through six stages in their process of change, each as important as the others; however, we personally would say that the second stage, Contemplation, or the beginning of conscious involvement in habit change, is the most important and probably most difficult. Contemplation is where, in order to get started with habit changes we desire, we need to identify our values and priorities and to recognize the internal voices guiding and persuading us toward our habitual behaviors.

The first stage, **Precontemplation (Not Ready)**, represents people who aren't intending to take any action and/or aren't even aware that they need to make a change because they don't realize that their behavior is problematic to them and, possibly, to others. Although identified as "a stage" in the model, this isn't actually a stage or step in change so much as an indicator of what exists before change begins. The second stage, **Contemplation (Getting Ready)**, represents people who become aware that their behavior in fact is problematic and begin to explore, understand, and discuss pros and cons of their problematic habits and to investigate the values and priorities that inform those habits. At the third stage, **Preparation (Ready)**, people are biopsychosocially prepared to begin their change within the next 30 days and, when they begin, to take small steps towards their goal(s), all along believing that change will improve their lives. During the fourth stage, **Action,** people intend to keep moving forward by modifying their problem behaviors or acquiring more healthful new ones. With the fifth stage, **Maintenance**, people have sustained their behavior change for at least six months, guaranteeing there will be no relapse. And with the last, sixth stage, **Termination,** people know and feel that they have no desire to return to their bad habits and no worry about ever personalizing them again.

TTM identifies its model as cyclical because progress as we develop behavior and habit change often is momentarily interrupted or prohibited by biopsychosocial factors requiring us to retrace or reinforce previous steps that originally had moved us forward. To be used at any stage in the Change Model, TTM offers "cognitive, affective, and evaluative processes. . of change [which] have been identified . . . result[ing] in strategies that help people make and maintain change" (TTM). We encourage you to think about each of these processes and, throughout your expedition toward change, to use any of them that best suit your needs and will promote your progress:

1. **Self-Liberation:** Your commitment to change behavior based on the belief that achievement of the healthful behavior is possible.

2. **Self-Reevaluation:** Realizing through self-reappraisal that the desired healthful behavior and habits are part of who you want to be.

3. **Dramatic Relief:** Involves emotional excitement and favorable stimulation about your current behavior and the psychological relief that can come from changing from Stage 1 Precontemplation to Stage 2 Contemplation.

4. **Consciousness Raising:** Increasing your intellectual awareness about the wellness behaviors you want to incorporate into your life to replace your bad habits.

5. **Environmental Reevaluation:** Social reappraisal to realize how your bad behavior and habits can or do affect other people.

6. **Stimulus Control:** Re-engineering the environment to have reminders and cues that support and encourage the healthful behavior and remove those that encourage the unhealthful behavior.

7. **Social Liberation:** Making attempts to decrease the prevalence of your former problem behavior in society. This can come through "counter-conditioning."

8. **Counter-Conditioning:** Substituting healthful behaviors and thoughts for unhealthful behaviors and thoughts, and possibly participating in environmental opportunities to support your improved behaviors, which in turn will empower you through new, changed behavior.

9. **Helping Relationships:** Finding supportive relationships that encourage the desired change.

10. **Reinforcement Management:** Rewarding the positive behavior and reducing the rewards that come from negative behavior.

Use these ten biopsychosocial processes whenever you return to the TTM to locate whatever stage requires attention to your immediate needs, and whenever you want to add to the self-helping strategies you learn as you continue through this chapter.

You can further develop your management and control of *The Power of Habit: Why We Do What We Do in Life and Business* by understanding Charles Duhigg's "The Habit Loop," which explains how bad habits have triggers or cues that provide short-lived rewards. Nicola MacPhail argues similarly and explains how this 'habit loop' can condition our behavior. In a response to a particular cue, MacPhail writes, you behave in a certain way. When that behavior or response feels good, you respond that way again the next time you encounter that cue. The more you respond that way, the less you think about it—and the more likely you are to respond again and again in the same way. This 'habit loop' of cue or trigger→response→reward is present in everyone, and as adults we perform habit loops conditioned in childhood that have informed our behavior whether or not we're aware of them. Important to know is that scientific studies suggest you're much more likely to fall into a habitual loop due to negative emotions. In fact. those emotions often become the cues or triggers to the habit's responses themselves; for example, people complain that they eat more when they're bored or tired. Others drink alcohol more or smoke when they're stressed. People procrastinate—in itself a bad habit—because they feel no joy about the task they face. MacPhail concludes by noting that much of our behavior, and our ability or inability to execute it effectively, is the result of our physiological and emotional needs and impulses. And, unfortunately, the habits that are linked to emotional cues are the hardest to crack. However, by being aware of what those cues are, you can intervene by replacing your responses.

This awareness, emphasized by MacPhail and Duhigg, is the second stage of TTM, Contemplation, and, as we said earlier, probably is the most difficult yet important part of behavior modification and habit change. To help you to promote your own self-awareness, here are five introductory questions you should ask yourself, suggested by Pete Lieb-man in "What Causes Bad Habits—And What Can You Do About Them?" These questions are intended to be general leads that you can follow as you initiate your inquiries into your unhealthful behavioral habits. As always, be honest with yourself as you reflect on your habit-ual behaviors and examine their causes and effects:

i.   Where are you when you enact or do your bad habit? Your physical environment can cue bad behaviors, such as a bar and drinking, work and junk food, living room and televi-sion.

ii.   Whom are you with—or are you alone—when the bad habit occurs? Examine your social environment, whom you're around, and, if any of the surrounding behaviors seem potentially contagious, consider if they've been likely to affect your own. For example, encouragement to "let loose" or "be free" is a contagious behavior; as a cue it also might trigger additional drinking, unnecessarily increased loudness, or "unwoke" physicality.

iii. How do you feel (physically, mentally, emotionally) when you enact your bad habit? When you're tired, which is a physical cue, possibly you crave ice cream. When you need to procrastinate, a mental cue, possibly you turn to social media online. When you're stressed, an emotional cue, pos-sibly you smoke "to relax."

iv.   What typically has happened immediately before you enact your habit? Possibly you eat junk food because just before you've argued with your spouse or child or colleague. Pos-sibly you explore social media whenever you want to avoid an immediate responsibility. Possibly you smoke or drink whenever you enter a social setting.

v.   Are there particular days and times of day when your bad habits are likely to occur? (Liebman)

Although it may seem that habit change is as simple as proceeding systematically through programmed stages, we all know that there always will be obstacles standing in the way of our behavior modification and habit change and preventing it from being easy—regardless of whatever kinds and degrees of success we've attained in the past. Remember: TT2's model is cyclical, allowing us to return to earlier stages whenever necessary, because significant behavior modification seldom progresses forward in a straight line. David discovered this truth most instructively when taking Precision Nutrition's amazingly profitable PN2 Coaching Certification as part of his diverse fitness training; its valuable biopsychosocial lessons helped not just himself as a coach, but his clients alike with an understanding of what must go into habit change and what the underlying roadblocks obstructing that change may arise from. As self-advertised, Precision Nutrition "is the industry's first comprehensive program of its kind—and the only one built specifically for health and fitness coaches to add a rare 'deep health' skill to their toolkits." This "comprehensive program" addresses not only nutrition as its focal center, but "the science and practice of better sleep, effective recovery, and more resilience to stress . . . [by] unlocking hidden stressors" (ttps://www.precisionnutrition.com/).

Beyond its certification's academics, Precision Nutrition has a masterful way of helping one understand how to begin the process toward change, illustrating the compassion and empathy needed to keep you focused even when you fall off the game plan. Since each person's values and priorities may differ, there is no "one size fits all" approach that will work with habit change. Change requires lots of digging in and research to find out each person's relationship with what needs to change, and why it needs to change.

As you read further, keep in mind the important word "relationship," used in the preceding sentence. Let's consider, as an introductory example, your relationship to the television, which we choose because most people have and watch a TV. Each of us has specific ways we interact with or relate to our TV, some of us to get information through the news, some of us to connect with people, to gather a family, to share a ritual such as eating with friends while watching a movie or a show. These relationships to the TV are great ways to use it; however, life isn't one-dimensional and we know there are flip sides to those "great ways," in this case maybe watching TV out of boredom, watching TV for companionship, watching TV when you're stressed, watching TV when you're angry or sad, watching watching watching. It's fair to ask why these latter ways of watching TV are a problem. The answer is because these ways of using the TV are more of a distraction and aren't done for a genuinely beneficial purpose, thus taking awareness and resolution out of our control and turning off our minds, as if that avoidance of our boredom, loneliness, stress, anger or sadness would bring us tranquility and rest. On the contrary, this is one of the main reasons why today's society has excessive health issues such as depression, anxiety, and obesity, to name only a few. In our experience, many of these health issues—and often they're triggered or cued by watching TV or other tech screens—can be resolved with awareness of and compassion for one's self. In the next few pages we intend to explain this, keeping in mind the important word we mentioned earlier: relationship.

While David was listening to Pastor Michael Todd and his friend Dr. Dharius Daniels discussing Relationship Goals, they said something profound: "Your greatest pleasure and greatest pain both come from the same place, Relationships." It struck David that although they were speaking about human relationships, this same principle applies to our personal relationships within ourselves and with everything around us, on a daily basis—in sum, our biopsychosocial relationships; those include our relationship with sleep, food, stress, vices, ourselves and how we view ourselves and, given how we view ourselves and our self-worth, very possibly our families, inner circle of friends, and work colleagues.

Comprehending the nature of our relationships leads us to better understand our values and priorities and, with that understanding, to modify any behaviors or change any habits that can damage us and others in our world. In one of his uncut videos, Pastor Michael Todd further states that you cannot have relationship goals if you do not have aim, and many times people do not have aim because they are looking at the wrong target. For biopsychosocial wellness or health, this theory can be applied similarly: you can't have wellness goals if you don't have the proper targets or markers that you're aiming at to change. With so many things that one can choose to focus on, what should today's society take aim towards? This is where the art of biopsychosocial wellness plus behavioral modification gets to apply its creativity, because each person not only has different values and priorities, but also has different susceptibilities and compensatory needs.

One of David's favorite terms that he learned while studying PN2 was "allostatic load," which explained exactly what had been weighing on him personally for so many years, driving some of his bad decisions and habitual behaviors that he couldn't control—but needed to control—for self-improvement. Introduced by McEwen and Stellar in 1993, allostatic load is the cumulative burden of stress from life events, more specifically "the cost of chronic exposure to fluctuating or heightened neural and neuroendocrine responses resulting from repeated or chronic environmental challenges that an individual reacts to as being particularly stressful" (Karger). Your body naturally responds to these stressors in an attempt to regain homeostasis (stable bodily conditions), but when environmental challenges exceed an individual's ability to cope, then "allostatic overload" ensues. Unfortunately, you carry this allostatic overload with you into everything you do in life, and therefore it influences many—possibly too many—of your decisions. This is why we think behavior change is about relationship management, which is how we interact with every component in our lives. If you want to do well in life, you really need to do well in relationships.

In many instances the allostatic load comes from your relationships with immediate family, possibly even extended family. It also can be society-driven: very often we look at what our current societal "norms" are, use them as reliable measurements and guides, and contrast our situations against these "standards." Understandable but nonetheless injurious, these societal norms may cause stress because of our perceived economic situation or our dissatisfaction with our employment; less defensibly, we rely on those standards to set the expectations we have for all the relationships in our lives. The unfortunate part of looking at these societal norms is that many times the snapshots of a moment that we look at, admire, and choose as our measurements and even our goals have neither historical nor future value attached to them; intangible mirages of desirability, they become meaningless when we try to actualize them. Instead of focusing on societal norms, we should focus on what we consider as being our actual flaws and then reset our values and priorities. Because "Habit protects us from anything we don't have a set way of handling" (Alsadir, 1), revocation of a bad habit requires a bigger awareness of self! And if you possibly can get better at knowing and being you, then we all possibly can get better at knowing and being us! Imagine a world in which all or most of its people were able to manage their allostatic load and had no overload driving their compromising and socially divisive behaviors.

In his book *Wellness Counseling,* Paul F. Granello defines wellness as "prevention or lifestyle-habit change"; further. he believes that "the future of professional counseling (and all helping professions) is going to be strongly related to prevention and wellness" (vii). Initiating habit change at any time in your life, because it's self-helping, therefore is a form of prevention as well. Applied to this idea of prevention, the "Highlights" section of the article "Pathways to well-being: Untangling the causal relationships among biopsychosocial variables" presents all six potential pathways among biological (B), psychological (P), and social (S) factors. All of these preventive relationships influence wellness and can potentially contribute to subjective well-being and to objective physical health outcomes—if we're aware enough to change our negative habits requiring alteration. In summary, the article explains that

> The influential pathways that lead to subjective well-being are S→P and B→P pathways, although these pathways can be impacted by psychological factors that differ among individuals. For objective health outcomes, the P→B and S→B pathways appear to be important, where the latter pathway is mediated by psychological factors. We additionally highlight the importance of systematically understanding subjective experience,

> which represents an epistemologically distinct domain, and describe how subjective experience can explain individual differences in causal pathways (Karunamuni).

Indisputably, overall health is an active state in which you must make constant efforts, in your environment, to achieve and maintain wellness and, logically, to prevent unwellness. You have a distinct group of biopsychosocial factors influencing your actions to attain overall health, and, frequently, certain kinds of habit-change are required before that total wellness can occur. What follows in three sections are 18 desirable targets to aim at for improved "relationships" decreasing your allostatic overload and leading to greater wellness. Grouped separately for your convenience, these three sections actually are inseparable, listing and exploring reciprocally reinforcing biopsychosocial behaviors and indicators. This list will help you further to recognize and to contemplate—Stage Two of The Transtheoretical Model—your values and priorities as actualized in your thinking and demonstrated through your behavior.

Bio[logical]

1.   Health Biomarkers

Biomarkers are measurable substances in humans and any other organism whose presence indicates disease, infection, environmental exposure, or post-treatment medical status; not symptoms, these biomarkers can be found through blood tests, x-rays, and CAT scans, and they are our best medical means of risk prediction or post-operative recovery. As an obvious example, high LDL cholesterol is a biomarker of cardiovascular risk. Investigating your health biomarkers will help you to know whatever potentially may be standing in your way for attaining wellness. Although additional studies are warranted, one study's 2003 results of eight published, randomized trials "suggest that biological information conveying harm exposure, disease risk, or impaired physical functioning may increase motivation to change" (McClure). Since 2003, many additional studies have found that physical activity, healthful eating, and emotional well-being do in fact improve if patients receive feedback about their personal biomarkers.

Begin by asking yourself if you have a family history of any type of disease. Do you have any current symptoms of disease that you have been diagnosed with? Have you been prescribed any medication(s)? Do you suffer from any symptoms of your health issues? Do you suffer from any symptoms of your medication(s)?

2.   Do You Listen to Your Body?

Are you aware that your body speaks and sends messages to you constantly? Did you know that your brain, in addition to receiving information from your five senses, receives information from the internal sense receptors located in muscles, joints, and internal organs? As any of your internally coordinated functions move away from balance and optimal function, your brain learns about it. It follows that these messages are feedback which, if listened to, can help you to determine if something's wrong with you and, if so, to identify the cause or source of that wrongness and, then, to restore balance. Restoration of your internal balances may need to come from habit change or modification of some of your behaviors.

The next three bio[logical] categories—Movement, Nutrition, and Sleep—are discussed at length later in this book; therefore, if you know you'll be needing to break any bad habits or to modify your behavior in the context of these three categories, then use whatever knowledge and self-awareness you gain here and apply it to the subsequent chapters.

3.   Movement

Do you exercise at all and, if so, how frequently do you exercise? What kind(s) of exercise do you do? Are you mostly inclined to lead a sedentary life? Do you have any injuries or orthopedic conditions that impede your ability to exercise? Is exercise difficult because of heart disease risk factors such as obesity, high blood pressure, high blood cholesterol, and type 2 diabetes? Whatever your situation and present level of activity, you can change it for improvement. Remember that Rome wasn't built in a day, and keep in mind the Chinese proverb that says, "A journey of a thousand miles begins with a single step." You may fear that first step because your goal for physical movement seems too remote, the distance to it impossible to attain. Yes, taken individually, each small step you take, were you to take it, may not seem all that significant; probably it isn't. Nonetheless, it's become part of a process leading to new levels of productivity. And when you add up each day's small step over time, cumulatively those steps can show discernible progress and lead to extraordinary results.

4.   Nutrition

It's remarkable that people don't connect the dots between how they feel and the foods they eat. Because food affects every body, everybody needs to understand the ways that insufficient nutrition can keep them down, hold them back, and limit their abilities to thrive and succeed as individuals or as a society. To move forward toward better nutritional habits, first develop your self-awareness by noting the foods and liquids you eat and drink, when you eat and drink them, the frequency with which you eat and drink in a given day, especially if snacking is involved, the quantity of food you eat at each meal, and an understanding of the quality of food you eat at each meal and over the course of the day. See the Big Picture of your food and liquid intake. Certainly it may help to consult a nutritionist to learn the qualities and acceptable quantities of your intake, but you easily can find nutritional values online if you want to begin on your own.

Next, discover if you're aware of your hunger cues. Are those cues natural and biological, thus true cues, such as your stomach growling, or low energy, shakiness from low glucose, headaches, and problems focusing? Or, conversely, is your hunger cued or triggered by psychological and/or social factors? Listen or sensitize yourself to these signals, so that in the future you'll recognize them for what they are and help you to decide if you're really hungry.

Last, are you aware of your satiety cues? Have you eaten slowly enough to allow your body time to let you know it's full? Even if you know you're full, do you continue to eat more because there's more on your plate? Is it possible that long-term stress, which floods your body with cortisol, a hormone that makes you want to eat more, is an ongoing state for you? If you're constantly fatigued, the likelihood of your eating more than you need also is hormonally triggered: your levels of ghrelin, a hormone that makes you want to eat, go up, while your levels of leptin, a hormone that decreases hunger and the desire to eat, go down, the result being that you feel hungry even if your body doesn't need food. Is it possible that when you feel nervous or anxious you're inclined to eat more? Do you experience peer pressure or less obvious social influencing to cause you to be excessive with drink or food during social gatherings? Have you ever experienced yourself eating simply because the food is there and easy to grab from your refrigerator or pantry? (Mikstas).

5.   Sleep

As with all the other biological factors discussed here, begin by surveying your sleeping habits and your relationship with them. How many hours of sleep do you get per night? How many hours of sleep do you get per week, if for example weekday nights provide less sleep, weekend nights more? How would you rate your sleep (Very Poor to Excellent) on a scale of 1-10? Are you a light or heavy sleeper? Are you affected by Sleep Apnea? Is your sleep disrupted frequently or infrequently? What causes the disrupted sleep?

Psycho[logical]

1.   Perfectionism:

Although the pursuit of excellence can be an admirable, healthful habit (it's always important to do your best when trying to achieve an important goal), keep in mind that habitual pursuits of perfection can become negative if you set standards beyond your reach, which means they're not "smart goals." Unhealthful perfectionism exists if you're dissatisfied with anything less than perfection, preoccupied with failure or disapproval, and habitually see mistakes as evidence of unworthiness. Additionally, when your perfectionism turns negative, it can escalate your anxiety and stress, and can tear down your healthful boundaries. When you're focused solely on being perfect with no boundaries on how to get there, it's easy to get lost. Many behaviorists advise practicing mindfulness to steer your perfectionism to the positive side; Ironically however, mindfulness isn't a clear concept, so let's just say that ruminating darkly about your own worth, skills, or prospects won't influence or change an inherently irrational voice; therefore, work to recognize your inner critic as nothing more than an entrenched bad mental habit, and shift your relationship with it. Create some distance from your inner voice of negative judgment.

2. Regret:

A possible consequence of perfectionism is the bad habit of regret, which, with daily practice, can turn into lifelong rumination—dark contemplation—over what might have been. Some people are wouldacoulda-shoulda regretfuls, whose habitual practice can lead to depression, anxiety, sleep problems, and difficulty concentrating. Creating those slowdowns, regret sometimes can inhibit forward movement and can even negatively affect physical health. The truth is that you can't go back in time and that, in fact, you didn't do what you woulda-coulda-shoulda done. So be it. Even if your decisions cause you pain and discomfort, they're only temporary. Don't cry over spilled milk.

We advise that you not think in absolutes: to believe that you have or had to make the right decision and that anything else is unacceptble is almost certainly setting yourself up for failure and unnecessary pressure. However, if you assess your decisions with the knowledge that you make thousands of choices each day and that human limitations prohibit you from getting all of them right, then you're more likely to make a decision knowing that you can endure the consequences. Change your habit of regret from the rigidity of right and wrong, of perfect and horrible, to a flexibility that allows you greater peace somewhere between those extreme opposites. You're just not going to be

100% satisfied after every decision in life, although regretfulness often makes you react as if you expect yourself to be. Know that there always will be "what ifs" and that sometimes—dare we admit it—we just don't have all the answers. Accept that you're fallible. Naturally there are different kinds and degrees of decisions to make, some of them having negative repercussions that can affect others if your choice proves to be poor or unwise. But keep in mind that making a bad decision doesn't make you a bad or incompetent person; you're still the same person. So take a breath, and remember that harping regretfully on a bad decision can lead only to a worse case of the coulda-woulda-shouldas.

3.   Guilt:

Guilt has a proper function in society, because recognizing causes for feeling remorseful about a wrongdoing usually prevents a person from committing that offense again. The habit of guilt often starts in childhood, when you learned to act a certain way out of fear that your family wouldn't be proud of you or that you'd be punished for "bad behavior"; as you grew older, the emotional grip of guilt may have matured too, because, as a person's ego forms in adaptation to the external world, the many "thou shalt nots" whose restrictions we impose on ourselves to be admired and accepted can bring embarrassment and shame if we find ourselves not abiding by them. Rational self-awareness helps to mediate this tension, but many people subconsciously allow guilt to well up within them and, as life develops and you age, bad habits of guilt can develop; these include the distorted magnification of problems, which in turn causes guilt; your claimed responsibility for creating or resolving problems that had little or nothing to do with you; your perceiving yourself as a bad person for committing minor offenses; and your refusing to forgive yourself.

Rational self-intervention can help you to avoid those negative kinds of excessive guilt by balancing ego with guilt, and by understanding behavioral limits that provide well-being—in effect, by processing guilt in a way that's actually productive. Because guilt comes up when there's a tension between your actions and expectations, you can examine your guilt honestly and change those expectations or change your behavior. You may feel guilty about leaving your family to go to work, for example, and then feel guilty about leaving your job to go home to your family. Left unchecked, you may find yourself in a state of perpetual guilt that prevents you from giving your full attention to any one task.

4.   Failure Mindset:

Self-doubt and negative thoughts can discourage you from setting smart goals, diminish the value of your natural talents, and magnify your missteps. To minimize your self-doubt, create a list of your skills, talents, and achievements, reading the list regularly to remind yourself of both your potential value and achieved worth and, when you hear the self-doubting voices in your head that say you cannot succeed, that you have no choice, and that you should back out before the world discovers you're a fraud, remind yourself of all the reasons you're "good enough." Another way of understanding the failure mindset is if habitually you put yourself down. It's impossible to perform well when you're telling yourself, "You're stupid" or "You can't ever do anything right." Negative self-talk will discourage you from putting in your best effort, and it will drag you down fast. Stop the put-downs: talk to yourself like a trusted friend, and be compassionate. If you wouldn't use such harsh words with someone else, don't allow your inner critic to say them to you.

5. Making Excuses:

Blaming other people or external circumstances for your lack of achievement harms your performance. Saying things like "My boss is holding me back," "All this paperwork makes it impossible to do my job," "Society sees me as being too old," "Not enough time exists for me to do this," or "I'm not getting support from my spouse and friends" will only keep you stuck. Stop making excuses: focus on all the things you can do rather than on what you think you can't because of external circumstances. When you pay attention to the positive, you'll put more effort into your performance.

6. Catastrophizing the Future:

Negative predictions about your personal and professional future easily can turn into self-fulfilling prophecies. If, when going to the gym, you presume you'll be inefficient, relatively weak, and won't last long, then it's very possible that you'll become distracted by that negativity, whose energy—all thinking is energy— will indeed help to downgrade your performance at the gym. If you have to give a speech at the PTA and believe that you're going to forget parts of it, then in fact you've increased the likelihood that you will. Break the habit of catastrophizing. Predicting disastrous outcomes will cause a spike in anxiety that could cause you to choke.

Psycho↔Social:

Most of the habits discussed previously, under Psycho, may not affect anyone but yourself, although certainly their impact can reach beyond you. It's likely that you'll privatize your self-help in modifying or changing those habits because you don't want them to affect anyone else's life and don't feel that they should be shared. In this psycho↔social section, however, you'll learn that some psychological habits inevitably spill out into social situations and that their damage can impact more than just yourself.

Four Horsemen of Relationships

All of us need to be aware of and to sensitize ourselves to the "Four Horsemen of Relationships" when we interact with other people. Taking a toll on whoever is involved, both the giver and receiver, the Four Horsemen are

- criticism
- contempt
- defensiveness
- stonewalling (giving or receiving the "cold shoulder").

While such habits may not seem detrimentally large-scale, they nevertheless can affect our and others' mental health and, taken to extremes, can even be classified as forms of emotional abuse (Lisitsa). Although modifying these bad habits may seem common-sensical, "Being able to identify the Four Horsemen in your conflict discussions is a necessary first step to eliminating them and replacing them with healthy, productive communication patterns" (Lisitsa). Again, important yet difficult to achieve, this identification, elimination, and replacement of these bad habits is what the second stage of TTM (the Transtheoretical Model) is about. Self-awareness is critically important if we are to effect change for self-improvement.

First, then, be honest: can you become critical, contemptuous, defensive, or a stonewaller in social or professional situations? After you've recognized that you have (≠ you are guilty of) any of these tendencies, begin to examine the contexts in which they're likely to occur. Bob, for example, still can be and in the past definitely was both critical and

84

defensive, so he's taught himself to recognize the cues or triggers that condition/ed his habitual critical and defensive responses. Now, when the cues occur, immediately he thinks of how to reformulate—and re-place—those two habitual reactions; over time, he's created better conversational habits.

If you're likely to parade any of the Horsemen, don't let them trample other people.

Social

1.   Stress Levels

Stress is a vast category, broad and deep, and it looms large whenever health professionals speak of wellness because its omnipresent influences of differing kinds and degrees do in fact impact on sensitive humans throughout each day, at every turn. The most major causes of stress include the death of a loved one, divorce, moving your residence, major illness, job loss, and economic insecurity, but stress in its steady streams can be caused by work, relationships, finances, health, and media overload. The Mayo Clinic tells us that "stress symptoms can affect your body, your thoughts and feelings, and your behavior. Being able to recognize common stress symptoms can help you manage them. Stress that's left unchecked can contribute to many health problems, such as high blood pressure, heart disease, obesity and diabetes" ("Stress Management").

True for all biopsychosocial factors pertaining to wellness, stress first must be recognized: you need to be aware of whatever and however stress affects you. Simple questioning can help: How stressed do you feel? What do you think causes your stress? When are you most stressed, and does knowing this help you to determine the cause? How do you deal with your stress? Keep in mind that all of us experience and process stress differently because all of us are different. Some people are worry-warts and drive themselves into stressed irrationality over mundane realities or possibilities. People obsessive about time may feel an inordinate amount of stress if immobilized in a traffic jam, or if late to a lunch with a friend. People determined to control their lives may become stressed when anything or anyone impedes that need for control; all unexpected variables in life weaken some people's need for control. Related to that need for control, stress can come with uncertainty; all of us on planet Earth felt stress because of Covid's unpredictability. Some people internalize large amounts of stress by watching the world's infuriating and gloomy news, or ruminating on dark subject matter. The yapping dog next door may cause you stress, or the honking horns and jackhammers on the street outside, or the way someone looked at you on the sidewalk—or even the pitch of someone's voice.

Self-helping cures for stress can come in many forms, all of which involve activity: exercise; relaxation techniques, such as meditation, yoga and deep breathing exercises, tai chi or massage; keeping and exercising your sense of humor; being around non-toxic family members and friends in enjoyable social situations; reading, listening to music, and engaging in hobbies, all of which remove you from self-focused tensions.

2.   Overuse of Social Media

According to The Pew Research Center, "69% of adults and 81% of teens in the U.S. use social media [undoubtedly those percentages increased during the pandemic]. This puts a large amount of the population at an increased risk of feeling anxious, depressed, or ill over their social media use," a conclusion corroborated by "a recent survey of 1500 adult Facebook and Twitter users in which 62 percent of participants reported feelings of inadequacy and 60 percent reported jealousy from comparing themselves to other social media users. Thirty percent said using just these two forms of social media made them feel lonely" (Sawarkar). And a 2021 study published in *Psychiatric News* further links the use of multiple social media platforms with an increased risk for depression and anxiety. Before you know it, with this kind of social media existence, you're second-guessing decisions you make, values you hold, and the validity of your goals because you keep comparing yourself to someone else's success; further, you subject yourself to needless emotional hurt and potential psychological damage. One possible mechanism accounting for this depression and anxiety "is that people who use many different platforms end up multitasking, such as frequently switching between applications or engaging in social media on multiple devices. Studies have found that multitasking is related to poorer attention, cognition, and mood. Other potential problems of using multiple platforms include an increased risk of anxiety in trying to keep up with the rules and culture associated with each one and more opportunity to commit a gaffe or faux pas since attention is divided" (Zagorski). But whatever factors work as causes for the conclusion that overuse of social media is a bad habit, the effects themselves confirm it. We can understand these negative effects elementally by using the psychological presupposition that most social media follows the Greater Internet Fuckwad Theory, proposed in 2004 by Mike Krahulik and Jerry Holkins, which says that when a normal person "is allowed anonymity and an audience, they lose social inhibitions and act inappropriately." In other words, "people become trolls on the internet because there is someone to pay attention, but no one to shame them" (Quora). What therefore can and does run rampant on social media are shaming, cyberbullying, and mental harassment and aggression.

3.   Overuse of a Smartphone

An absence of good news in notifications, a steady stream of distressing news coverage, and fighting on social media can amplify negative effects of smartphone overuse. Bad smartphone habits include constant checking to see if you've been contacted; reading or texting while you're walking or driving; consequent inattentiveness to your surroundings, including its natural beauty and architectural magnificence; relying on your phone's GPS, which limits your own navigational abilities, spatial sensitivities, and sometimes common sense; substituting calls or texts for interpersonal human contact; even using your phone in public restrooms, as has been true the multiple times that we've seen and heard men speaking on their cells at office and gym urinals. And speaking of urinals: did you know that phone screen surfaces are dirtier than toilet seats? Yes, our smart phones now seem indispensable to our normal daily coursing of affairs and management of life's many duties. Nevertheless, it may be time for a digital detox, a modified removal of yourself from your relationship with our cell.

༺ ༺ ༺ ༺ ༺ ༺ ༺

All of us are creatures of habit, some of those habits biologically natural and unvarying. Our autonomic nervous system, for example, controls the function of our organs and glands, as well as our reflexes; it confers with our Circadian rhythm and winds our biological clock, which beats and ticks habitually, as does our heart. We sweat to control body temperature. Babies suck their thumb as soon as no nipple is available. In countless ways, we humans are hardwired to exist with certain kinds of autonomic habits, a bodily truth. Psychological hardwiring, however, is another story. Nigel Nicholson tells us that recent convergent theories from research and discoveries in genetics, neuropsychology, and paleobiology have been brought to light by the new field of evolutionary psychology, which posits that although human beings today inhabit a thoroughly modern world of space exploration and virtual realities, they do so with the ingrained mentality of Stone Age hunter-gatherers. *Homo sapiens* emerged on the Savannah Plain some 200,000 years ago, yet according to evolutionary psychology, people today still seek those traits that made survival possible then: an instinct to fight furiously when threatened, for instance, and a drive to trade information and share secrets. Human beings are, in other words, hardwired. You can take the person out of the Stone Age, evolutionary psychologists contend, but you can't take the Stone Age out of the person.

If you don't agree with the preceding quotation, then you're like many academics still involved in the ongoing nature/nurture debates concerning human behavior. And those who dispute the quotation will argue that so much of what we do with habit-breaking is an attempt to take the Stone Age out of our behavior, or at least to modify it. That Stone Age "drive to trade information and share secrets," for example, may be what inclines many people to be gossipy; however, social ethics inclines lots of those many to work to break or modify that habit.

Setting aside whatever innate drives may or may not exist in human nature—and we encourage you to set them aside, as you can go in endless circles about the essential nature of human nature—we in fact also live according to humanly manufactured routines that breed habits. The impositions of time and its schedules regiment much of our daily movement and impose regularities upon us. We behave with high levels of repeated activity within similar contexts, as putting our mobile phone onto charge when coming home from work and mixing a drink or pouring a glass of wine. We live in standardized sequences or routines commanded by logic, such as brushing our teeth after we eat. Some of us rely on specific steps of a certain "proper" order, first this, then that, always the same, such as habitually putting on our socks before our pants, or vice versa. Some of us eat the same foods bought at the same stores, typically sit in the same seat at the dinner table, use the same barber or hair stylist, follow the same ole, same ole. Some of us won't step on sidewalk cracks or walk under a ladder, superstitious habits.

We safely can conclude that internally and externally the clocks of our existence inform and regularize our lives, with habits whose developed frequency often supplants what we'd like to think is our freely willed behavior. The beauty of free will, however, is that its subversion can be reversed by itself, and indeed we can plan and think to eliminate bad habits by knowing what they are, becoming aware of how they affect our behavior, and working to modify the cues or triggers that have conditioned us to react or respond in detrimental habitual ways. To the extent that you have free agency in the directions of your life and the management of your behavioral inclinations, therefore, we encourage you to add as another fundamental of biopsychosocial wellness the elimination of what you know to be your worst habits inhibiting your best self.

WORKS CITED

Alsadir, Nuar. "Clown School," *Granta*, 31 October, 2017. https://granta.com/ clown-school/

Bryner, Jeanna, "Bad Habits; Why We Can't Stop," January 11, 2008. *Live Science.* https://www.livescience.com/1191-bad-habits-stop.html

Duhigg, Charles, *The Power of Habit: Why We Do What We Do in Life and Business.* New York: Random House Trade Paperbacks, 2014.

Gardner, Benjamin and Amanda L. Rebar, *Habit Formation and Behavior Change.* King's College London: January 2019. https://www.re-searchgate.net/publication/330406744_Habit_Formation_ and_Behavior_Change Granello, Paul F. Wellness Counseling. Boston: Pearson Education Inc., 2013.

Karunamuni, Nandini, "Pathways to well-being: Untangling the causal Relationships among biopsychosocial variables." Social *Science & Medicine*, 10, February 2020.

Liebman, Pete, "What Causes Bad Habits?" *StrongerHabits.com*

Lisitsa, Ellie, "The Four Horsemen: Criticism, Contempt, Defensiveness, and Stonewalling." The Gottman Institute, April 23, 2013

(https://www.google.com/search?q=%E2%80%9CThe+four+horse-men+of+relationships&ei=W3eqYZCJFuSbptQPt-bqk8A4&ved=0ahUKEwjQovfdtcj0AhXkjYkE-HTUdCe4Q4dUDCA4&uact=5&oq=%E2%80%9CThe+four+horse-men+of+relationships&gs_lcp=Cgdnd3Mtd2l6EAMyBQgAEIAEMgY-IABAWEB4yBggAEBYQHjIFCAAQhgM6BwgAEEcQsAM6BQgAE-JECOgUILhCABDoOCC4QgAQQsQMMQxwEQowI6CA-gAEIAEELEDOgsILhCABBDHARCvATDNEpUTHQoQUJMHL-rErGJyHg89uy71MyuHABBCxAxCDATDNEpUTHQoQUJMHL-

rErGJyHg89uy71MyuHILhBDOgsILhDHARCvARCRA-
joKCC4QxwEQowIQQzoECAAQQzoICC4QsQMQQI6BQguE-
JECOgglABAWEAoQHkoECEEYAFDJHliXcmCodGgBcAJ4AYABxg-
GIAd0akgEEMzYuNpgBAKABAcgBCMABAQ&sclient=gws-wiz)

MacPhail, Nicola, "What Causes Bad Habits—And What You Can Mac-
Phail, Nicola, "What Causes Bad Habits—And What You Can Do
AboutThem"

McClure, Jennifer, "Are biomarkers useful treatment aids for promoting
Health behavior change? An empirical review." *American Journal of Preventive Medicine*, 2002 Apr;22(3):200-7.

Mikstas, Christine, "Why Do You Eat When You're Not Hungry?"
NourishbyWebMD
 https://www.webmd.com/diet/obesity/ss/slideshow-why-eat-when-not-
hungry

Rosenthal, Samantha R. et al., "Negative Experiences on Facebook and De-
pressive Symptoms among Young Adults." Jonson and Wales University:
2016

Sawarkar, Ananya, "6 Things That Could Damage Your Mental Health."
Psych2Go, July 23, 2021.

"Stress Management," Mayo Clinic.

https://www.mayoclinic.org/healthy-lifestyle/stress-management/in-
depth/stress-symptoms/art-20050987

Thrive Global

https://www.google.com/search?q=causes+of+bad+habits&ei=jVCmYf-
HEArXmxgG89owAQ&ved=0ahUKEwixv_CUwMD0AhU1szE-
KHTz7AxYQ4dUDCA8&uact=5&oq=causes+of+bad+hab-
its&gs_lcp=Cgdnd3Mtd2l6EAMyBggAEAcQHjIGCAAQBxAeMgUIA-
BCABDIGCAAQCBAeMgUIABCGAzI-
FCAAQhgMyBQgAEIYDMgUIABCGAzIFCAAQhgM6BwgAEEcQsAM6

BAgAEA06CAgAEAgQDRAeOggIABAIEAcQHkoECEE-
YAFDHGVimOmD3SmgBcAJ4AYABTYgB2QSSAQIxMJgBAKABAc-
gBCMABAQ&sclient=gws-wiz

Zagorski, Nick, "Using Many Social Media Platforms Linked With Depression, Anxiety Risk." *Psychiatric News*, 17 January 2017
https://doi.org/10.1176/appi. pn.2017.1b16

https://drhyman.com/blog/2010/12/31/the-failure-of-decoding-thehuman-genome-and-the-future-of-medicine

https://www.karger.com/Article/FullText/510696

https://www.precisionnutrition.com/

https://www.sciencedirect.com/search?qs=habit%20change%20and%20

biopsychosocial%20wellness

CHAPTER IV

Before Trauma Hits:
Avoiding the Worst Habits

Dr. Rob Curran

"Without commitment, you'll never start, but more importantly,
without consistency, you'll never finish."
- Denzel Washington

Hi, I'm Rob. And I have bad habits, which allow me to make decisions which I regret at the end of the day or sometime in the future. I invite you to examine the two top charts on my desk on any given day.

Patient A: a 75 year-old woman who had fallen while going from the bedroom to the bathroom. Her x-rays and CT scan reveal a hip and pelvis fracture, as well as bleeding in and around the brain. Her history reveals that she is on medications for osteoporosis, high cholesterol, high blood pressure, gout, arthritis, and "blood thinners" to prevent the blood clotting, which could cause a stroke.

Patient B: a 57 year-old male with an infection, cellulitis, in his lower leg. He has been diagnosed with Type 2 diabetes mellitus for over ten years, has a lifelong history of obesity, and takes medication by mouth for his diabetes.

Without my assigning blame or having a crystal ball, many of the conditions which cause us so much pain, stress, shame—and did I mention BILLIONS of dollars in medical costs and unproductive days—are somewhat self-inflicted. Let's look at the first chart a little further, which presents an older adult who fell, a very common occurrence. A fall from standing height which results in hip and pelvic fractures is commonly associated with the bone-loss disease osteoporosis, and muscle loss, known as sarcopenia. In 2019, 34,212 older adults aged 65 and older died from preventable falls, and over 3.1 million were treated in emergency departments. Over the past 10 years, the number of older adult deaths from falling has increased 58%, while emergency department visits have increased 34%. But, osteoporosis doesn't sneak up on you like a sniper. While it is true that bone loss is higher in women after menopause, in this patient menopause was likely twenty or more years ago. Was she monitoring her bone health? Did her New Year's Resolutions include strengthening her bones and muscles every year?

Muscle mass loss is an age-related condition and one of the physiologic changes involved in sarcopenia. Muscle mass loss has a cause-effect relationship with muscle strength. Loss of both muscle mass and strength increases with age and is a problem for the elderly since it can result in a poor quality of life and in physical disabilities. Muscle mass loss can be caused by various factors, including disease, decreased caloric intake, poor blood flow to the muscles, a decline in anabolic hormones, and an increase in pro-inflammatory chemicals. Weight loss is also associated with the development of muscle mass loss. In addition, studies have shown that aging is associated with a physiological loss of appetite that leads to weight loss. Loss of hormones, such as testosterone, DHEA, and growth hormone occurs with aging. People with diabetes mellitus have accelerated muscle loss. Stroke and hip fracture are highly prevalent among the elderly and usually rapidly lead to an increase in muscle loss. This appears to be due to disuse and inflammation, stroke, and/or denervation.

The prevalence of muscle mass loss is increasing and is expected to continue to rise in the years to come. 5-13% of people 65 years and older have low muscle mass; the percentage increases up to 50% in those over 80 years old. By the age of 80, an estimated 40% of the muscle mass present at age 20 is lost. Currently, sarcopenia affects more than 50 million people worldwide and is expected to affect 200 million individuals in the next 40 years.

Bone mass loss is a condition known as osteopenia. Osteopenia often progresses to osteoporosis, a condition characterized by the reduced bone mineral density and increased rate of bone loss. Bone mineral density decreases with age. Therefore, the probability of a person suffering from osteopenia or osteoporosis, and related skeletal fragility, increases with age. The causes leading to bone mass loss are multifactorial and similar to the causes of muscle mass loss. The most common cause of osteopenia is aging. Skeletal aging is known to progress faster in women than in men due to hormonal changes after menopause. It is estimated that the number of adults over age 50 in the United States with low bone mass, including osteoporosis, is 64.4 million. By 2030, that number will further increase to 71.2 million. It is anticipated that the number of fractures will grow proportionally.

What can you do?

There are a number of strategies to prevent further bone and muscle loss. Muscle can even be GAINED at every age tested so far under the correct supervision and coaching. But, such tests need to be done wisely, in consultation and collaboration with experienced medical professional(s) to prevent injury to bones, hypertensive and cardiac complications, and even death. All of these strategies begin with a comprehensive medical examination performed by a professional with experience and expertise; note that this might not be your regular primary care physician. Talk to your doctor or medical provider about your concerns so that you can be referred to an appropriate specialist and that your records can easily be transferred and discussed. Physicians who truly work with patients to reverse muscle loss and stop bone loss most often have completed a residency or fellowship in sports medicine, preventive medicine, physical rehabilitation, or women's health. A physical therapist or exercise physiologist should also have advanced certifications and experience in the prescription and supervision of exercise programs, specifically to reverse muscle loss and maintain bone strength. Prescriptions for restorative hormone therapy and bone loss agents may be considered based on the results and monitoring of blood tests.

Adequate nutrition, especially protein intake, is the cornerstone of reversing muscle loss and preventing bone loss. Reducing food intake in the older adult has consequences that could be important for muscle mass and strength. Reduction of energy intake corresponding to lower levels of energy consumption leads to weight loss and, ultimately, to muscle mass loss. Proteins provide the necessary energy source for muscle protein production.

Strength training using adequate and appropriate resistance has been shown to be effective to combat the loss of muscle mass. Regular weight-bearing and muscle-strengthening exercises can reduce the risk of falls and fractures. This type of exercise can increase the bone density as well as the strength by micro-architectural bone arrangement. A 6-month Tai Chi program was shown to be effective in decreasing the number of falls, the risk of falling, and the fear of falling, in addition to improving functional balance and physical performance in physically inactive persons aged 70 years or older.

Maybe our 75 year-old Patient A thought it was too late for her?

As the economy and society have changed over time, so have our habits. We are more sedentary. Less than 5% of adults participate in 30 minutes of physical activity each day, and only one in three adults receives the recommended amount of physical activity each week. Both of the patients above could have benefitted and could still benefit from an appropriately prescribed exercise program. In one study, people with Type 2 diabetes exercised for 175 minutes a week, limited their calories to 1,200 to 1,800 per day, and got weekly counseling and education on these lifestyle changes. Within a year, about 10% got off their diabetes medications or improved to the point where their blood sugar level was no longer in the diabetes range, and was instead classified as prediabetes. Results were best for those who lost the most weight or who started the program with less severe or newly diagnosed diabetes. Fifteen percent to 20% of these people were able to stop taking their diabetes medications.

Diabetes results in active years lost, earlier heart attacks, strokes, and dialysis. Our habits can prevent it and even reverse it in early stages.

Our habits, what we do every day, define us. To understand a poor food choice habit is not to just say, "I overeat," or "I eat too much sugar," or "I had pancakes at 2 a.m." One has to see there are psychological, emotional, societal, and other pressures at work in all of these habits, biopsychosocial influences impacting on wellness. Some people are "stress eaters"; that is their nature, their brain sending calming, relaxing signals only when it receives signals that the stomach is filling with food. What fills the stomach quicker: bacon, egg, and cheese on a bagel, or carrots? How did emotion play into that person's mind when they were shopping? What does the instant gratification of a pizza delivered at any time do to your brain's regulation and impulse control? These patients don't need a lecture on healthful eating; rather, stress eating is almost an unstoppable force.

I have read that a man named Isaac said that an object that is at rest will stay at rest unless a force acts upon it. Every personal trainer, physical therapist, and cardiologist will agree. Physical activity is almost as complicated as eating. There are psychological factors at play, such as the camaraderie of team-sports, especially when picked up at an early age, which can help a child fit in, develop relationships and a peer network of other "athletic" people to whom physical activity becomes second nature, and is enjoyable. The other side of the coin is the person who goes to a gym or facility and has to "work it out," where it is a task. They may be great at 100 different things, but none of them involve sweating for a half-hour or more several times a week.

Brain Biology

There are a few select chemicals in the brain that are important to this discussion. One is dopamine, known as the feel-good neurotransmitter—a chemical that ferries information between neurons. The brain releases it when we eat food that we crave or while we have sex, contributing to feelings of pleasure and satisfaction as part of the reward system. This important neurochemical boosts mood, motivation, and attention, and helps regulate movement, learning, and emotional responses. You may already be familiar with dopamine from the condition Parkinson's Disease, which is a profound loss of production of dopamine.

Much of our understanding of habits and brain chemistry, while still rudimentary, comes from observing how much dopamine is produced when a test subject does something. We know that dopamine is released when the light on your cellphone blinks or you feel/hear the vibration. Any parent of a current teenager can argue that there is a cell phone habituation/addiction, and every teen can probably argue that their parents are just as addicted.

Habits-Anonymous

Alcoholics Anonymous and organizations that have followed in its footsteps have saved countless lives by providing a support group and in some cases accountability for people. Did you know that there was no science or evidence in planning the "Twelve Steps"? There were 12 steps because there were 12 Apostles of Jesus Christ. Be that as it may, how many of us could use the support offered by a 12-step program to help develop better, healthier habits?

For many people it is the New Year's Resolution to lose that weight, get in shape, get to the gym, drop the bad habits. According to one non-scientific study, by January 12 a majority of the group reported they had broken their "resolution." Many of those resolutions regarding health have to do with trying to turn back the hands of time. We want to lose some weight we have gained over time so our knees, hips, and back don't feel so sore after a regular day that the thought of exercise makes us cringe. We want to still be attractive to our partners, or maybe we are looking forward for a new relationship.

How are our habits formed? First, you pair two things together, a stimulus (food) and a response (salivating). Stimulus (food) results in Response (salivating). Then you add an additional stimulus: Stimulus 1 (food) + Stimulus 2 (bell) results in Response (salivating). Over time you will be able to remove the original stimulus, and have just the additional stimulus elicit the response: Stimulus 2 (bell) results in Response (salivating). As a real-life example of this,

Let's look at smoking:

Stimulus 1 (seeing cigarette) results in Response (light up and smoke the cigarette). Then we add:

Stimulus 1 (seeing cigarette) + Stimulus 2 (feeling bored) results in Response (light up and smoke the cigarette). Until we get:

Stimulus 2 (feeling bored) results in Response (light up and smoke the cigarette). Keeping this original research in mind, let's explore what we now know about creating or changing habits.

1. Small, specific actions are more likely to become habitual.

Writing down you want to lose 50 pounds by July is ludicrous. Or you will be able to do 50 pull-ups. Cross that off as a resolution. Let's discuss the habits that will result in….um.. results! Let's start small. Assess your average day. Are you very sedentary? Is your idea of exercise walking up the steps to the train each morning? Let's change that. Let us start small, but impactful, perhaps "I am going to walk from home to the supermarket and back every day after work (if you have dogs, bring them along; they'll love it!). The walk to the supermarket is probably not going to result in weight loss, but you are laying the foundation for a habit. After this has gone on a while, now you have scheduled maybe a twenty-minute or half-hour opening in your day to walk to the supermarket and back. With that, now you might be able, instead of walking to the supermarket, to add that you are going to watch an exercise video on Youtube for free, a low impact exercise tape. Further, now your arms and legs are moving. And after a while you can say . . . maybe, I'd like to try this kickboxing or higher impact video (I want to sweat some more). You started with making a relatively small commitment, but it carved out time in your life, and look at you now: every day after work your routine includes 30 mins of kickboxing, or multi-joint high impact exercise, getting you sweating and your heart rate elevated.

Perhaps you are working from home or at an office. What can you accomplish with 5 minutes an hour in an office or in your home office/school? Would your heart benefit from some increased blood flow from marching in place for just five minutes each hour? Not a race, just movement. When you move, the joints you are moving self-lubricate. Marching in place moves blood and fluid out of your lower legs, moves the big muscles in the front and back of your legs, and helps the ankles, knees, hips, and low back stay loose and healthy. After an 8-hour day, you will have marched in place for over half an hour.

Maybe you are reading that Keto diets or Paleo diets or whatever the flavor of the day is will cause weight loss. But, you love your pasta, or you live near THE BEST pizza place in all of Brooklyn. The likelihood of your maintaining that no-pizza diet is nearly zero. So what can you do? Now, again, we need to look at ourselves, this time examining our eating habits. Keep a journal, maybe take a camera pic, or keep a video diary of everything you are eating and why. Were you truly so hungry just three hours after a bowl of lasagna that you needed 8 chocolate chip cookies? Maybe you were, maybe you just saw those cookies and your brain lit up its happy hormones for you. So, maybe, can you have just a half-bowl of lasagna (or just one slice instead of two slices of pizza)? Come back tomorrow for the other slice. Can you break that one habit of having 2 slices of pizza at a meal? Trust me, your brain will be having an earthquake eruption: "THERE'S ANOTHER SLICE THERE FOR ME." But leave it for tomorrow. Over a period of time, your body and brain will get used to just one slice. After a period of time your body and brain will get used to you having only five beers of a six-pack, throwing the last two cigarettes out with the empty pack, etc.

As you start on this journey … what are your goals? Do you want to stop shopping at the Big & Tall store? Do you want to go from XXXX clothes to XXX, to XX, to XL? Is there a waist size you remember as an adult that you want to target? Maybe you haven't seen your toes in a few years? Maybe you don't want to have so much leg pain? Maybe you want to be able to bounce your grandson without breaking out in a sweat? Know first what your habits are, and then set goals that include NOTHING RADICAL!

Substantial weight loss is possible across a range of treatment modalities, but long-term sustenance of lost weight is much more challenging, and weight regain is typical. In a meta-analysis of 29 long-term weight loss studies, more than half of the lost weight was regained within two years, and by five years more than 80% of lost weight was regained. Indeed, previous failed attempts at achieving durable weight loss may have contributed to the recent decrease in the percentage of people with obesity who are trying to lose weight, and many now believe that weight loss is a futile endeavor. It follows that "I will lose ten pounds this month after giving up pizza and alcohol" is more than likely a foolish commitment. Instead, give yourself a comprehensive review of when and why you are eating. Can you really not wait for your dinner at a restaurant without an order of potato skins or mozzarella sticks or buffalo wings? Isn't that a bad habit, appetizers before a feast at a restaurant or diner? Here we encounter loads of opportunities to make good choices. Mashed, baked, or French fries? Soup or salad? With Dressing? Something smothered in cheese perhaps? Well, maybe, but hopefully not again this month.

On medical forms it says to ask about "Sleeping Habits," because we all have our own routine. We know this can be negatively affected if we have guests, or if the kids come in and kick around, or our work schedules change, and for a period of time our brains and bodies will struggle to get back to our baseline. But, eventually, we will reach a new normal.

I'd rather read these:

Patient A: a 75 year-old came in for her annual physical. Last year's exam revealed bone loss and muscle loss. She also needed medication for her high blood pressure, gout, arthritis, and "blood thinners." She led a sedentary lifestyle, occasionally going out to meet friends or meet at the senior center. Her exam reveals that she has not lost any bone since last year, has gained 8 pounds and 5% of her muscle mass. She can do several push-ups and barely complains of arthritic pain. She joined a Tai-Chi club and does Tai-Chi online for 45 minutes twice per week. She has a serving of protein with every meal. Her blood pressure is down from 150/94 last year to 138/80 now, a dramatic improvement reducing her likelihood of suffering a stroke. She has moved away from the status of "pre-frail" to "not-frail."

Patient B: our 57 year-old male, also presenting for his checkup, has been diagnosed with Type 2 diabetes mellitus for over ten years, has a lifelong history of obesity, and takes medication by mouth for his diabetes. His average blood glucose last year was 285, his blood glucose at today's visit is 130. He has lost fifteen pounds from his visit last year, and gone from a size 44 waist to a size 38 waist in pants. His New Year's Resolution was to "sweat every day for 25 minutes," which he did, on most days. After meeting with his doctor for clearance he began walking up and down the stairs from the lobby to his second-floor apartment. First, he started only when there were commercials on during his shows, then it continued to "during halftime" of his sports shows.

Don't end up as one of those sad self-defeated charts at the beginning of this chapter. There are healthful habits you can make right now to change your future. Put this book down and walk, wheel, crawl to a destination of your choice! DO IT NOW!

CHAPTER V

Neuro-Orthopedic Pain Management
Luke Bongiorno

Your brain is a lawyer, and a really good one at that. Your brain will rationalize its behavior based on what it thinks is the truth or credible evidence. For example, when you feel pain, your brain will try to convince you that your shoulder is bad, or your posture is poor, or your hip is weak, presenting a case to yourself against your shoulder, posture or hip. But what if you overwrite those thoughts and present a case to counteract the pain? What if you start to think, "My shoulder is secure, my posture is good, my hip is strong"? What if you reframe your thoughts to convince yourself that you can function healthfully and without pain?

This leads to some fundamental questions about the nature of pain:

What exactly is pain?

What is the biology of pain?

Why do people feel pain?

Why does physical and emotional pain get mixed up?

How is pain managed at different stages in life?

In essence, the modern understanding of pain is that the brain decides when it occurs. For example, if you're walking across a busy highway and stub your toe, you're less likely to feel pain because there are cars moving back and forth and you have to concentrate on running to safety. But if you stub your toe with the same level of force at home in the middle of the night, you'll experience more pain. Why? Because pain is related to the context in which it occurs; perception of pain depends on the momentary balance between danger and safety. Pain exists when the lawyer-like brain finds more credible evidence of danger to the body than it does safety. Conversely, pain does not exist when the credible evidence of safety is greater than the credible evidence of danger. The brain constantly assesses all the perils going on around you, creating pain episodes according to its perception.

Luckily you are not your brain, and your brain is not you. We are much more than just our brains, and our brains can be trained, usually with the help of more information from a trusted source. Our brains can therefore adapt and change via a process known as neuroplasticity. Presented with new information and/or experiences, the brain can effectively release a body part from a pain episode.

To manage pain, instead of looking at the body as a biomedical tool in separate parts—shoulder, elbow, wrist, etc.—it is more holistic to assess the body from a biopsychosocial standpoint in which biological, psychological, and socio-environmental components intersect. As healthcare professionals we can provide evidence and educate patients to help them understand that everything, every body part, every thought and emotion, every environmental experience, is connected. And this knowledge gives the patient permission to look at pain and injury objectively, and not from a place of fear.

The biopsychosocial framework and a reminder:

Pain involves the intricate variable interaction of biological factors (genetic, biochemical, etc.), psychological factors (mood, personality, behaviour etc.) and social factors (cultural, familial, socioeconomic, medical etc).

107

INTERSECTING BIOPSYCHOSOCIAL GRAPH

When working with a new pain patient, the first step I use to evaluate them and unlock their mind-body-pain connection is to share the benefit of looking at the person as a whole. I help them understand how their systems integrate and function and assess the areas of their body and their life that are in and out of balance. Not just physical balance, but also the balance of their mental and digestive wellbeing, and how it all interrelates. As a healthcare professional, by not directly addressing the painful part of the body per se, I'm helping the patient re-center their equilibrium to treat the whole system first. Depending on the age of the patient, their willingness to accept the mind-body-pain connection will vary, so we must adapt the approach accordingly.

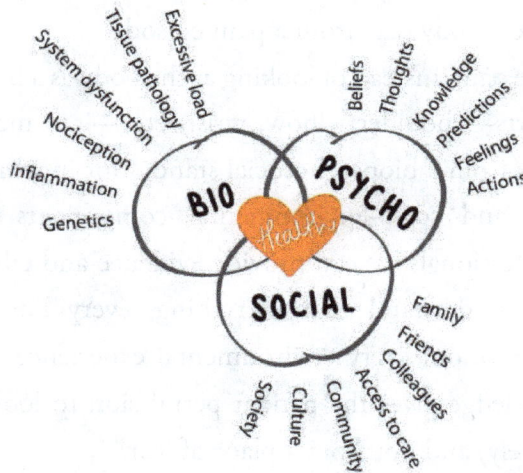

AGE & WISDOM

Young high school and college students are often open to new ideas. They want to learn. However, they look good, they feel good, they perform well and so are less likely to end up in the office in need of pain management. But when they do, they are easy to work with. You can educate a student.

While millennials are often similarly openminded and willing to learn, they can sometimes be a little more challenging. They know their bodies but they don't necessarily understand the mind-body-pain connection. They are confident and tend to challenge authority when something doesn't fit their paradigm of thinking. When educating millennials that there are alternate, more holistic ways to treat pain, care must be taken with both words and tone to avoid unsettling such individuals and potentially limiting their learning.

Those aged 40+ want to stay in their 40s for as long as possible; it's like they're investing in a 401(k) for the body—thus reducing healthcare costs. For the most part they've worked very hard for a long time. They are tired, perhaps single, married, or in a relationship, may have kids, and have taken on a lot of responsibility managing emotional and personal relationships. This naturally creates stress or manifests itself in the physical body as pain. Their outlet is running, walking: whatever brings most satisfaction. They want to play golf, they want to play tennis, and they're more emotionally ready to hear about abstract ideas, maybe incorporating yoga and Pilates into their otherwise hardcore sport regimes. Seeking advice from healthcare professionals, they are ready and willing to listen, learn, and invest in their future health.

Every age group struggles with the aging myth. Twenty-five-year-olds think they're 'quarter-century-old,' while 45-year-olds are consumed by 'not being 25 anymore.' Likewise, the 65+ group are still in a battle against the aging myth. Their bodies are aging but, in many cases, their minds are young. They still feel like a 40-year-old. They might also think about something their doctor has said that has resonated with them, but which can also inhibit their recovery and progress. For example, if their doctor determines the injury is "bone-on-bone," then the idea that their knee joints are rubbing together can reduce their motivation to move. People in this age group tend to rely heavily on traditional medicine, but what if traditional treatments are actually holding them back?

If someone is feeling pain, a traditional doctor usually sends them for an MRI. What if people stopped getting MRIs? A tear might not necessarily be causing the pain, and surgery might not necessarily increase the mobility needed to get them back on the golf course. Instead of getting the MRI and discovering the tear, what if they just learned about their body, how to stretch, breathe, recalibrate and move? They might still be playing golf at 75. Or older.

BALANCE

When patients have pain or have been avoiding the use of a body part because they might have a break or a tear, their body's center of gravity, or the brain's ability to trust that side of the body, is reduced. For example, if you've had pain in your left leg for six weeks, your brain no longer trusts the information coming from that leg. The result might be that your muscles tighten a little more on the left, which means less of your foot is touching the ground, possibly resulting in having less feedback from the foot telling the left side what to do. Furthermore, if your brain is not trusting the information from your left side, you might put more weight on the right, so that you don't fall over.

When we are off balance, our sensory system is heightened. All of a sudden, something that doesn't normally hurt starts to hurt, creating a hyperactive response (allodynia). Something that might hurt for a few seconds becomes startling (hyperalgesia). When we are in balance, the same stimulus doesn't elicit the same response, so we feel less pain. Instead of our system being hypersensitized and, in effect, so overprotective that it won't let you move, it will be just protective enough. When the whole nervous system is better balanced, a more accurate read of what is actually painful and what is not becomes possible.

Balance is a combination of three things:

Proprioception, our body's ability to know where it is in space

Vision, use of our eyes to see where we are and acquire visual feedback

The Vestibular System, our spatial orientation, located in the inner ear.

All three work together to retain balance and can be utilized to manage pain. Let's imagine your vestibular system, feeling off-center in the inner ear, screaming, "Hey, you're leaning to the right!" In order to maintain the body's equilibrium, this prompts your vision to take over. You might feel as if you're in balance, but your perceived center of gravity, instead of being dead center, has shifted a little to the right. People are often unaware that they are off balance, until, perhaps, they close their eyes.

Vision not only is important to balance, but is also a very important way to objectively "look at" and assess the pain in question. For example, our brains recognize big scars or a lot of blood as pertinent visual information, giving such past and present damage a lot of attention and most likely triggering a heightened pain reaction. This was demonstrated in a study published in the *British Journal of Medicine* in 1995 in which a person was taken to the emergency room in excruciating pain from a nail that had gone through his shoe and foot. The doctors took off the shoe and realized that the nail had actually gone between the second and third toe; it hadn't even pierced the skin! The pain the patient was experiencing was interpreted not by what he felt, but by what he saw. The visual information carried more weight and had more influence in what we call the "pain neurotag"– the group of neurons that light up when we have a pain experience.

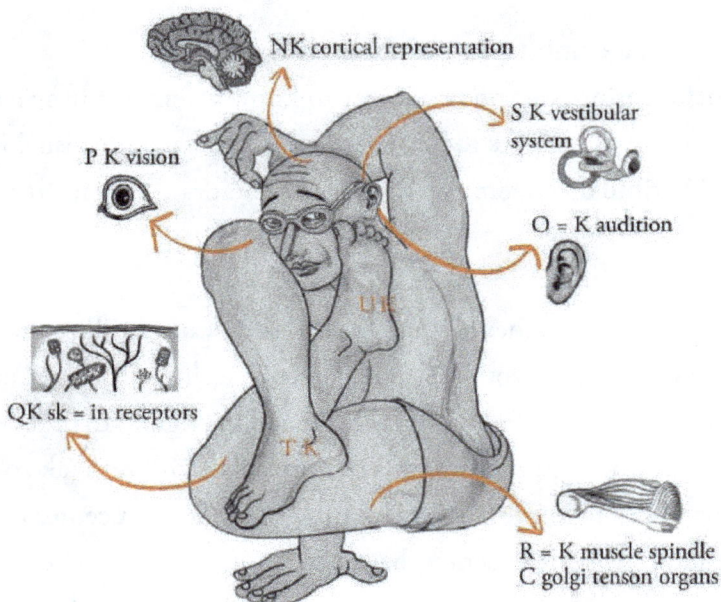

A widespread network of cortical brain areas is thought to be involved in body representation and, thus, in self-localization. However, a major role is also played by audition (2) and vision (3). In order to locate one's body part, both skin receptors (4), muscle spindles and Golgi tendon organs (5) are crucial. Together these cues contribute to create a unique and coherent percept of one's own body, well described with the concept of cortical body matrix. In particular, the innovative aspect is the body-centered representation of the body itself (instead of a body part-centered representation) such as the right leg (7) usually in the right side of the space (8) can occupy the left side of the peripersonal space simply crossing over in the space where the left leg usually is.

MENTAL WELLNESS

Anxiety is essentially the fear of the unknown and can be heightened when we feel pain in our bodies. Knowledge, combined with trust, can help re-write painful patterns, and help calm the mind and nervous system. By closing our eyes, looking inward, and doing visualization exercises, we can help mitigate a pain experience and calm the nervous system. In essence, the mind is our drug cabinet, which when calm and collected can release powerful antidepressants. Guided meditation is a great way to trick our minds into forgetting about pain. Within our brains we have a homunculus, which is basically a circuit board where each body part is represented – hands, feet, hip, spine, neck, and so on. When people who have had a leg amputated experience phantom limb pains, it is because their leg is still represented in the brain within that "circuit board." When you have an injury, the corresponding part of the brain gets bigger; it gets inflamed and disturbs connections to other body parts, so even when you don't have pain, you are still thinking about the injury: "Is my hip going to hurt me?" Doing exercises and practices such as guided meditation can broaden attention to the other areas of the brain, effectively to the other body parts. This helps to normalize the homunculus, taking the magnifying glass off the hip. When the patient doesn't think about their hip as much, their nervous system calms down and they start to feel better.

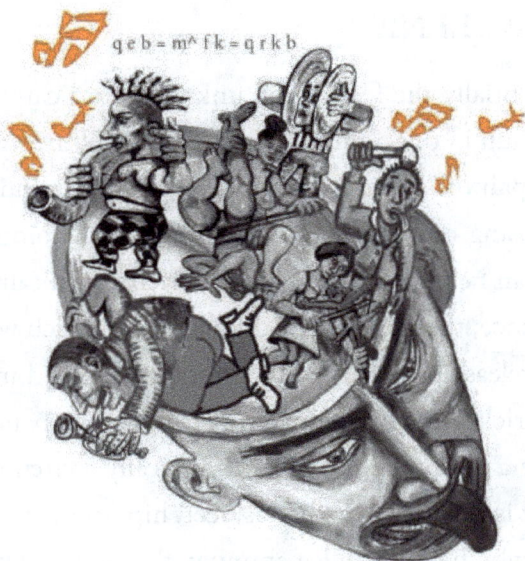

qeb=m^fk=qrkb

What if I have a stress fracture and I'm running through that pain: how do I know if I'm doing too much damage? If I adopt a strategy, such as guided meditation or focusing my mind and my stride to a metronome, and the pain goes away, then I can say, "You know what? I'm engaging the rest of my body and I feel good!" Teaching people that they can control how they feel, their level of protection and their ability to move, just by changing the way they think and perceive pain, is not just mind over matter. I'm not making this up; we're actually creating biological shifts.

DIGESTIVE WELLNESS

We are what we eat. The gut microbiome is our second brain. It regulates the immune system, which is our defense system. During a stress response the immune system ignites, activating and releasing chemicals that create real inflammation. If the body perceives danger, swelling can occur without the presence of an infection (neurogenic information).

It's a sign the body is readying itself for whatever might happen. Furthermore, gut health is linked to the autonomic nervous system to determine whether we are in a sympathetic "fight or flight" paranoid state of thinking (everyone is out to get me), or a parasympathetic "rest and digest" chill state (we're all connected, everybody loves us and has our best interests at heart).

When we have a healthy digestive tract, we're digesting and eliminating toxins. If those toxins are not being cleared, or we're not getting good blood flow to our gut, or we don't have healthy bacteria, studies have shown that this can lead to mental health disorders. Anxiety manifests in the sympathetic nervous system. The toxins trigger the gut to send messages up to the brain saying, "I'm in danger, I'm under threat." Under these circumstances, someone might say something to us that causes us to personalize it and jump to conclusions. But if we have a healthy microbiome, we're not getting as many danger messages. We are in a chill, relaxed state and our level of reactivity is less. If someone says something mean, we think, "Huh, they must not be having a good day." We don't take it personally. We can connect and empathize more and are less likely to be affected.

It is common in many cultures to practice gratitude to prepare the body for receiving food. Giving gratitude or thanks before each meal helps to activate the parasympathetic nervous system and enables better access to that "off switch." So too does slow, deep diaphragm breathing (in for four seconds, out for six seconds) before diving into a plate of food. In theory, we are getting into a relaxed or reduced cortisol state and enhancing serotonin and dopamine, which allows the calm, self-regulatory system to monitor more accurately—to be able to determine I have or I haven't had enough.

As a healthcare professional, gaining insight into a patient's digestive health is a window into understanding their pain and anxiety and a pathway to their healing, as well as another opportunity to educate.

RIGHT JUDGEMENT

Words matter. Different emotions, different words, different people or different things can trigger a stress response within all of us, which can result in heightened pain.

By becoming more aware of the brain's role in pain, we can counteract the misconceptions of pain with strategies that challenge us to pay more attention to other body parts. By doing so, we can change what we think and believe about pain, come to a decision about what to do, and, ultimately, calm the nervous system, alleviate anxiety, and reduce pain altogether. The patient needs to believe they can heal. Belief comes from listening and trusting their body, not from their clinician's words. I may show you an exercise and ask you to mimic my behavior, and you might be apprehensive because your doctor said not to, or "Dr. Google" advised against it.

But here is a health professional whom you've developed a relationship with, who has helped you before and you trust, giving you permission to move. This permission gives you just enough courage to take yourself through a range of motions that you wouldn't normally feel comfortable doing. And not only do you actually not feel pain, but you actually feel better!

Once we believe and trust in ourselves, we can then exercise Right Judgement: our ability to make an informed decision based on our knowledge and understanding of what we can and cannot do. This is a major step because in a state of anxiety people have a tricky time making decisions. So if we understand what is going on, and we're in a calm state, our ability to make rational decisions is enhanced. This training alleviates the panic. Clarity of mind allows a more informed choice and Right Judgement to be exercised. Should I play tennis or not play tennis? Should I go for a hike or not go for a hike? When we have the information and we've been given permission to move, then we can make a better choice. We think, "I'm starting to feel this, I can work through it," or "Should I seek advice now?" Ultimately, we make better decisions.

PATIENT AUTONOMY

Two recent patient stories give prime examples of the teachable transition to patient autonomy.

Patient A just turned 80-years-old. Never planning to retire, he was married to his desk until Coronavirus hit and he was forced to stay home. Like most people his age, fear of the virus, coupled with the universal fear of getting older, forced him to limit activity outside the home; a sedentary lifestyle can speed the aging process. But most older people can do a lot more than they think—and Patient A was no exception.

He adapted to his "new normal" by participating in Zoom training sessions three times a week. Without having any physical interaction, he has lost 20lbs and is now able run a mile without pain around the lower loop of Central Park. He does his stretches, keeps active while safely distancing himself from others, and maintains a positive outlook on life. As a newly minted octogenarian, he is in better shape now than in his seventies. This is an example of someone who has essentially gotten younger, and who is open to being even better at 90 instead of thinking, "I've just turned 80, I'm on the downhill slope." The sky's the limit!

Patient B is in the 40+ age group, generally healthy and active.
When quarantine hit, she decided to challenge herself to 30 days of
yoga and fell in love with it. Thirty days turned into 60, and then zero
when her back and hip started to really bother her. She was also hiking
in Central Park almost daily but was in too much pain to continue.
Disheartened, she reached out to me for help. Her dialogue went something like this: "I love yoga. I did it 60 days in a row. It's supposed to
be good for me, but it hurt me. I knew it was too much. I knew I
should've taken a break, but I didn't. I love it so much, but now I can't
do anything."

Her mind and body were suffering, but she didn't know what to
do. She was beating herself up. Yoga, a positive, became more of a negative. She was spiraling downward. To her surprise, the first thing I
did was give her permission to keep moving, to keep at the yoga and
walking. By gaining permission from someone she trusted, she had the
little bit of courage she needed to feel like she could take the proper
steps back to health and normalcy. Then, I had her do a balance exercise
to assess her vestibular system. With her eyes closed, I had her march
on the spot, and to her surprise she turned 90 degrees without realizing
it, indicating that her balance system was a little off. To counteract that
I had her do some cognitive tasks including math and spelling. Since
the neurons involved in a pain experience have other functions, the
cognitive tasks light up the brain and basically hijack or override the
pain, as if switching on a bright light, to help reset the balance system.
We then did a guided meditation, drawing her attention away from the
back and hip and evenly towards different parts of the body. We next
did a seated breathing exercise targeted at stretching and strengthening
her hip flexor muscles and posture. By breathing into the diaphragm,

more oxygen floods into the tissues, which in turn feel safer and less painful. We downloaded a metronome app on her phone for her to listen to when she walks, ensuring that her stride and placement of the foot on the ground was even and level, giving her an external focus, which can also help reset the brain. Patient B recorded all of these instructions and referred to them daily; the pain went away. When the pain occasionally crept back up, just a quick check in with these tools was all that she needed to alleviate the discomfort and get back on track.

Patient B's new dialogue went something like this: "I'm starting to feel that pain again, so I'm not going to do yoga every day this week; instead I'm going to do it four days. Or I'm going to do some stretching when I'm walking, or, instead of doing a full yoga practice tonight, I'm going to do only a few sun salutations. I will pay attention to my feet and breathe more, so I'm not putting myself at risk. I am in control." She is now exercising her Right Judgment. As she, and all of us, become more mindful, our senses become more reliable and allow us to identify and address pain objectively before it becomes unbearable.

REFRAME THE PAIN

As healthcare professionals, our job is to build people's self-confidence and belief in themselves, and it is our responsibility to do so by educating patients in as honest a way as possible. Depending on the patient's age, physicality, mental and digestive wellness, and pain need, we use different language and different techniques to provide them with the knowledge and tools to assess their pain and manage it. We're not just providing physical therapy, but a combination of mental and physical therapy to treat the body as a whole.

I love the wisdom of the popular saying: Give a man a fish and you feed him for a day; teach a man to fish and you feed him for a lifetime. By reframing the patient's approach to pain, essentially we are teaching them to 'fish,' that is, how to care for their health without being reliant on others. It's then the person in pain's responsibility to acknowledge and work towards their goals if they want to maximize the effectiveness of their intervention and get the greatest return on their health investment.

If you feel pain, you have pain, but there are many ways to guide your system out of it. Knowing, understanding, wisdom: it can be that simple. Gaining knowledge is not learning; it's just acquiring knowledge. Learning is the active process. Once you've done the work, once you see and feel the positive results, you have experienced learning and seen change. You now have the wisdom to present your case and reframe your pain, releasing it, letting it go. You can confidently make decisions based on what's best for you, because now you are the expert on your own pain.

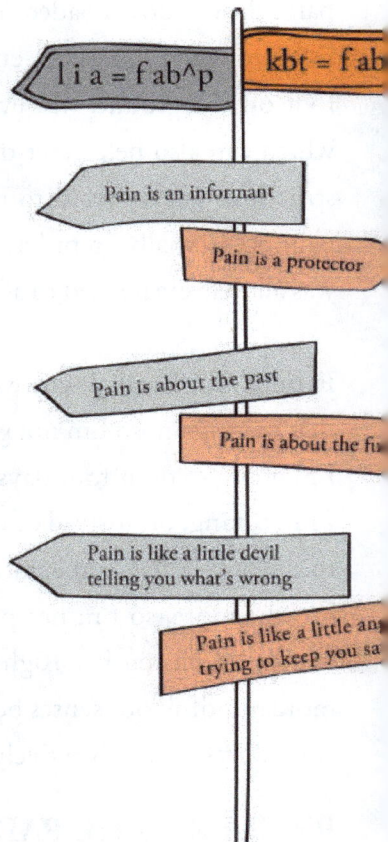

Sign posts (right side of page):
- l i a = f ab^p
- kbt = f ab
- Pain is an informant
- Pain is a protector
- Pain is about the past
- Pain is about the fu[ture]
- Pain is like a little devil telling you what's wrong
- Pain is like a little ang[el] trying to keep you sa[fe]

CHAPTER VI

Chronic Pain
Sam Visnic

What Is Chronic Pain And How Does It Differ From Acute Pain?

Put simply, chronic pain is pain that exists after the expected time of healing for an injury or ailment. While there is some disagreement on this, generally it works for our understanding.

We are familiar with acute pain, which is short-lived, and is often associated with an injury like a muscle strain, tear, or even a broken bone. These types of injuries heal in a fairly predictable amount of time, but if the pain persists past that time, the pain can be considered chronic. Most experts agree the majority of ailments in the body improve within a maximum of 6 months. If you're experiencing ongoing pain after 6 months.

It's a safe assumption you're now experiencing chronic pain. In this chapter, we will focus on chronic pain. The outcome is to give you a better basis from which to understand this type of pain. This better understanding can help you change the way you frame or think about pain, therefore changing how you respond to it, and potentially improving the results you achieve with various therapies. Learning about pain itself IS therapeutic!

How do people get stuck in the vicious cycle of chronic pain?

Approximately 20% of people will develop chronic pain, even if they do not experience an initial injury to their body! This is a staggering statistic, and one that sparks a lot of curiosity since it challenges the most common views on the nature of pain. While there are many factors that can contribute to the development of chronic pain, including genetics, and it's likely a perfect-storm type of scenario, there are a few observations that experts have noted with both the development and perpetuation of it.

Overemphasis on visual imaging

It is fairly well established that visual imaging such as MRI and X-ray don't tell the whole story when it comes to uncovering the root causes of pain. "Structural evidence of a lumbar disc hernia in a patient with appropriate symptoms is present more than 90% of the time. Unfortunately, even when using advanced imaging techniques such as myelography, CAT scans, or magnetic resonance imaging, the same positive findings are also present in 28% to 50% of asymptomatic individuals" (Leibenson, 76). Given this, you can imagine how common the diagnosis may purely be based on a visual scan, which may or may not align with the symptoms the person is experiencing. Not only leading to the wrong recommendation of therapeutic options or surgical procedures, it can also introduce unnecessary fear or concern in the pain sufferer, generating a serious concern over their situation.

Excessive focus on structural diagnosis and subsequent treatment failure.

This is associated with what was mentioned previously, but also takes into account the myriad of structural or movement diagnoses that are often found repeated online and/or in social media. This can include postural imbalance, muscles imbalance, faulty movement, weak core, etc. While some of these areas may include elements that can contribute to the overall pain experience, they are not the only factor by far. Excessively focusing on these areas often leads to missing more important factors that can be directly contributing to the development of the chronicity of the pain.

Every time a new diagnosis is received, and subsequently, the treatment fails to meet the expectations the person has, this leads to increased likelihood of developing a chronic pain issue.

Overlooking precipitating factors such as anxiety and/or depression

"Lindsay and Wyckoff found that up to 85% of patients with chronic pain fit the diagnostic criteria for clinical depression. Interestingly, it has also been found that 39% of patients with chronic pain have a history of depression that precedes the onset of pain" (Leibenson, 557). Anxiety and depression are very common amongst individuals who suffer from chronic pain. They can be associated with the increased likelihood of developing chronic pain, and certainly can be a product of experiencing chronic pain as well.

Influences like workplace injury and job satisfaction

Research has shown that pain treatment outcomes can be negatively impacted depending on the relationship of the individual to their work. People who are injured on the job are often faced with at least some disincentive for improvement, for they typically receive worker's compensation benefits, including medical coverage and financial benefits in the form of supplementary income, while avoiding the rigors of actually working for such benefits (Occupational Hearing Loss, 17). In some studies, researchers have concluded that compensation is related to increased reports of pain and reduced treatment efficacy. The results of meta-analyses suggest that this relationship is likely causal, and Rholing et al. statistically demonstrated that if compensation were eliminated as a variable, the experience of chronic pain would decrease by an average of 24% (Occupational Hearing Loss, 18). It's clear there are multiple factors that can certainly contribute to the development and perpetuation of chronic pain that must be uncovered.

Knowing Your Pain and Why It Matters

Approaching all pain the same way is a mistake. Using the wrong tool for the job will almost always end with a poor result. The type of pain someone has must be identified as closely as possible to know where to focus attention and what types of therapeutic elements or treatments will likely be most effective. Norman Doidge, M.D., eloquently writes about two people's success in chapter one of his new book, The Brain's Way of Healing: Remarkable Discoveries and Recoveries from the Frontiers of Neuroplasticity. Because the brain can reshape neural pathways devoted to chronic pain, pain occupies a mysterious place in medical terminology and diagnosis. Getting our heads wrapped around pain can be challenging. For the sake of brevity, it helps to put pain into a few simple categories.

There are three main categories of pain, and here we discuss the first two of them prior to the third. Knowing the type of pain helps us understand the best way to approach it. Most common ongoing aches and pains people experience fall into these categories. Most of us are familiar with the kind that arises from damaged tissue. Sprain an ankle, tear a muscle, that's nociceptive pain you are feeling. Damage in tissues triggers a response to send nociceptive input to the spinal cord and brain about the state of the tissues. It's important to note that nociception is not pain, just information. Nociception and pain are not equivalent, and there are no "pain fibers" or "pain receptors" specifically dedicated to relaying pain signals in the brain or body. Our nerve systems constantly send data to the brain for consideration about innumerable stimulating things like hunger, thirst, revulsion, desire, and pain. Pain, like all of the other sensations we feel, is, technically speaking, a brain-generated experience. Acute pain that is "in our body" like a broken ankle is meaningful and functional. Without the nervous system response and the brain's interpretation, we'd keep right on going and injure ourselves further.

The more sophisticated type of pain that occurs from damage to the system that reports and interprets injury itself to the nervous system is called neuropathic pain. If the peripheral nervous system is damaged or malfunctioning, called neuropathic pain, the brain is getting the wrong information, and pain changes accordingly.

While the nervous system is adapting to and reshaping the messages that we usually call pain, we experience different aspects. Neuropathic pains include phantom limb, neuralgia, carpal tunnel syndrome, and similar conditions. With nociceptive pain, the brain is getting the right information, but in neuropathic pain, the nervous system is damaged or malfunctioning. The brain is interpreting that information differently.

The most straightforward way to understand the difference is to imagine that you dropped your computer. You might have some dents and dings and a cracked screen, or your motherboard might have been damaged, and the machine will not work or will work poorly. So, you see, it's not just the tissues, nerves, or brain by themselves, but the interaction between these elements that can affect the pain experience.

There are different categories of chronic pain, and while it's possible to fit neatly into one or another, most people are split between these two categories to some degree. The more accurately you can determine where you stand, the more likely you can figure out the best way to address it. In the next paragraph, we discuss the third category and get at the root of more complex chronic pain conditions.

The third type of pain is called central sensitization. As we've discussed, the therapeutic establishment has been preoccupied with the structural and biomechanical causes of pain. Therapists are limited in their ability to treat some types of chronic cases successfully. By necessity, more therapists today are learning to treat their clients by incorporating an expanded model of pain that includes neurological and social definitions. It may be useful to frame our definition of pain as less of a negative. Pain is not a bad thing—pain is our primary alarm system. Just as you might assume that your house is being broken into when the home alarm goes off, pain necessitates our attention. We have to get out of bed, walk around the house, and see if it's an intruder or if the wind blew open the back door because someone forgot to lock it. The alarm did its job; it is up to us to pay attention and respond appropriately. To carry the analogy further—if we become overwrought with despair every time we hear a noise, we'd drive our spouses crazy. Conversely, if we don't investigate the door that won't close properly, perhaps we risk a home invasion. The same goes for pain: when we are consciously afraid of pain, or misunderstand pain, or otherwise try to ignore this natural, protective alarm system, we invite confusion.

The cycle of overreacting to the alarm system or misinterpreting the way it works is precisely how a patient becomes more sensitive. When a patient experiences more pain with less provocation, this is called "central sensitization." This term refers to changes to the central nervous system (CNS)—in particular, the brain and the spinal cord. Sensitized patients are more sensitive not only to things that may hurt but also to ordinary touch and pressure. Their pain also "echoes." These signals fade more slowly than they do in other people. In more severe cases, extreme oversensitivity is obvious. The role of sensitization in several common diseases has been proved and well documented, and it can also persist and worsen in the absence of disease and without apparent provocation. The neurological cascade of physical and mental experience is a complication of pain, also referred to as "chronicity." Central sensitization is the most common denominator in all difficult pain problems. It's nearly a universal factor that puts the "chronic" in chronic pain. Regardless of how it got started, central sensitization is the cause of its chronicity. The existence of central sensitization is quite well established, and yet there is a gap that exists in our scientific knowledge. There are no clear criteria for diagnosing central sensitization.

There is no easy laboratory test or checklist that can confirm it. It could be present in nearly any severe case of chronic pain. However, the pain could still be coming from a continuing problem in the tissue, with or without central sensitization. When central sensitization is suspected to be a strong contributor to a person's pain, therapists must adjust their methods. Central sensitization can easily be made worse by careless, deliberately rough, "no-pain, no-gain" treatment. When physical therapists, massage therapists, and chiropractors treat a chronic pain patient too intensely, they trigger the alarm system and make the person more sensitive, usually leading to more pain. Patients going through the "therapy grinder" often find themselves in the hands of overly intense therapists who are not familiar with central sensitization. Patients waste time, money, and precious energy on expensive and ineffective therapies only to find themselves crippled by pain and, sadly, depressed.

Care for chronic pain starts with normalizing the nervous system. Vigorous therapy can exacerbate a less serious problem and disturb the whole system easily. Early in treatment, patients with stubborn pain problems may start to feel that they are experiencing "too much" pain

—more than seems to "make sense." It's not an easy question to answer. When we hurt, our pain needs a voice. Like the patient with oversensitive hearing (hyperacusis) trying to figure out if sounds are too loud or just sound that way, pain can overwhelm the brain's ability to process it accurately. Essentially, when the nervous system is overly sensitized, and pain levels seem much higher than they may be, we need to be cautious when applying therapies that are painful to implement, such as deep pressure massage and even rigorous exercise. Tissue pathology that does not explain chronic pain is overwhelming (e.g., in back pain, neck pain, and knee osteoarthritis). Purely biomechanical explanations for pain are not helpful, so it's best to make sure any professional you see is aware of central sensitization. This is a solid criterion for choosing a therapist. If your doctor or therapist doesn't know what central sensitization is, it's likely best to take your pain elsewhere.

Keep in mind that you might go through quite a few professionals before finding one who shows "sensitivity to sensitivity." Keep in mind that even though medications that work on the central nervous system are the most promising treatment for severe pain system dysfunction, only a physician trained in the care of chronic pain can prescribe them. The best place to look for such a doctor is in a pain clinic. If you have persistent and severe pain, start looking for one today.

A note: regardless of whether or not central sensitization is happening in your body now, it always makes sense to be kind to your central nervous system. Make your life "safer" and less stressful. Gentler. Easier. Pain is not an "all in the head" problem, but a "strongly affected by the head" problem, such as an ulcer caused by a genuine bacterial illness and then severely aggravated by stress. When your CNS is "freaked out" and over interpreting every signal from the tissues as more painful, it's best to step back and let the body rest and reorient itself. The ability of the brain to form and reorganize certain synaptic connections, especially in response to learning or experience following injury, is known as neuroplasticity. The brain intuitively modulates excitability and neuronal activity when we are injured or distressed. Central sensitization is a modulatory process in the brain akin to a persistent state of high reactivity. In this state, the pain threshold is lower, and individuals may still feel pain after an injury has already healed.

In cases of nerve injury, both mechanical and chemical, the first alarm of peripheral sensitization is perceived by the brain as a constant, and it morphs into central sensitization. At this point, the initial pain signal is experienced as "louder." Central and peripheral sensitization may be responsible for various forms of pain that cannot be explained by a biomechanical model. The specific type of anxiety triggered by central and peripheral sensitization has two main characteristics— hyperalgesia and allodynia. Hyperalgesia is an exaggerated perception of pain after a stimulus that is mildly painful, such as slight pinpricks. Allodynia refers to experiencing pain with a stimulus that is not usually painful, as in simple touch or gentle pressure; however, individuals experiencing unexpected or random shifts in pain sensation are not making up their symptoms.

The same goes for those who sometimes experience improvements after taking medications, from physical movement, or from therapeutic massage. Diagnosis of central or peripheral sensitization is problematic. There is no laboratory test for this. How do we assess whether central sensitization is an actual diagnosis or a sort of syndrome that comes along with certain kinds of chronic pain in some but not all patients? This is a difficult question to answer, and in time, hopefully we will learn more about this, but one thing is certain in the meantime: A multidisciplinary, biopsychosocial- based TEAM approach is best when it comes to working with chronic pain to cover as much territory as possible.

The Biopsychosocial Model And Its Application To Chronic Pain

Until recently, the medical establishment tended to lean on a purely biomechanical description of pain that often fails to treat the whole person effectively. This leads to chronic pain sufferers, often experiencing a dizzying array of explanations for their condition. When we focus too much on biomechanical aspects of pain, we run the risk of ignoring the social and psychological issues of discomfort. This can feed into nervous system sensitivity and provoke further pain.

We know, for instance, that multiple inputs interact and contribute to a person's experience of pain. You will recall that pain falls into two primary categories. We discussed nociceptive and neuropathic pain. The former is associated with a specific injury, and the latter is a condition or disease in the nervous system. Adding a third category—central sensitization— provides a fuller explanation for more complicated pain cases. Most practitioners agree that it is best to focus on the whole person, not just on the area where the pain is. Person-centered therapy is unique. For it to be successful, it requires a thorough screening. Practitioners screen for biological, psychological, and sociological (biopsychosocial) factors and other health issues. If this is done well, we can identify the biopsychosocial factors that influence pain and disability.

It's necessary to communicate clearly with the individual to identify potential biopsychosocial drivers of pain. These include beliefs about pain, emotional coping responses, social context, and physical and other lifestyle factors. Chronic pain sufferers need to know how to confront how much their pain impacts their lives as a whole, the ability to work, interact socially, and positively integrate with society. This style changes the dynamics of the health practitioner-client relationship to "patient-centered communication." Naturally, if someone is suffering from chronic pain, they want to know that their health care provider cares about them by building rapport and connection to understand them rather than just treating them as a statistic, which unfortunately is the collective experience many people have in the current medical system.

Slowing down and taking the time to fully understand the scope of the person's issues, how it's affecting their lives, and getting details on the presentation of the pain can help build an alliance between the therapist and client. Research shows how powerful this alliance is when it comes to therapeutic success. An initial screen might include the following types of questions:

1. What is your pain story?
2. What do you think is the cause of your pain?
3. What do you do when pain increases?
4. Please tell me how your symptoms affected your ability to engage with functional and physical activity.
5. Do your symptoms worry you?
6. Why do you think you should not bend/lift/run?
7. What is your home/work/social life like?
8. What are your goals?

The answers to these questions can then guide an examination that explores the client's concerns, functional limitations, and physical capacity linked to their goals. I have found this dialogue to be of critical importance to many people. Often, clients will report that a considerable part of their improvement occurs when they feel their specific circumstances are addressed, rather than being given a generic approach based on their diagnosis, or condition. Thus, we are addressing the person, not the pain or biology itself.

This model was initially developed in 1977 by George Engel and is referred to as the Biopsychosocial Model (BPS). Since the biological aspects of pain are often over-emphasized, let's consider the psychosocial aspects of the BPS model. Psychosocial elements are profoundly impactful on an individual's health and, as we will discuss, their pain. A great deal of research has been done in this area, especially as it relates to issues such as back pain, which affects a large percentage of the population. When we become more aware of the impact of these elements, it becomes easier to understand why chronic pain sufferers may not respond to traditional nociceptive-based interventions. In the psychological aspect, there are some prevalent emotions that coincide with chronic pain. "Depression, anger, anxiety, and somatization (i.e., high pain sensitivity) are four broad emotional categories that have frequently been cited in the literature as being prevalent in the lives of patients with chronic pain." It's unclear in some cases if these elements are stemming from chronic pain, or preceded it, but consider this: "Lindsay and Wyckoff found that up to 85% of patients with chronic pain fit the diagnostic criteria for clinical depression. Interestingly, it has also been found that 39% of patients with chronic pain have a history of depression that precedes the onset of pain" (Morris, 557).

This is exceptionally high when you consider that the CDC says about 9% of Americans report feeling depressed on occasion, and about 3.4% suffer from major depression. Anger can be present in a number of different ways: the individual may be angry at their employer or some individual precisely for what they believe to be the cause of their pain; they could also be angry at their healthcare provider or their insurance company for the quality of the care they have been receiving; additionally, the individual could simply have a history of being a type of person that tends to be more angry or aggravated. No matter the cause, the presence of heightened levels of anger have been shown in some cases to lead to poorer pain therapy outcomes. Anxiety tends to exacerbate pain via activation of the sympathetic nervous system. This leads to increased muscle tone, fatigue, and thus more pain. Anxiety seems to go with the territory when it comes to chronic pain, and understandably when exposed to the biomedical model. It's easy to see how someone can become fearful of their "tissue issues" and become stuck in a seemingly endless loop of failed treatments, avoidance of activities, deconditioning, more fear, loss of hope, and thus more pain.

Waddell et al. identified a set of five "nonorganic signs" (the so-called Waddell signs) that can indicate a patient is being strongly influenced by factors other than the nociception generated by damaged tissue. Marital and relationship stress can be a significant factor in the chronic pain client as well. The ways in which spouses, family, friends, coworkers, and strangers respond to a person with chronic pain will have a tremendous impact on that individual through processes such as reinforcement and punishment. The role of relationships in chronic pain is very complicated. Pain may be serving the individual in their ability to have diminished functions in household and/or childcare duties, or income production. It can also be the opposite: their perception of their inability to perform in these roles may be exacerbating their stress and increasing pain. The role of the therapist is not to address these various psychosocial factors directly, but it is appropriate to educate the client on them, as well as validate to the client that these issues may exist, are genuine, and are indeed crucial in the overall therapeutic approach to resolving their pain experience. In both educating the client and validating their experience as usual as far as pain goes, we can effectively assist in reducing fear and anxiety, and thus improve the likelihood of a successful outcome in their pain therapy program.

Using a multi-disciplinary approach to address all aspects of the Biopsychosocial model No one can be an expert on everything, and each area can be addressed to start, but identifying which factors may need a deep dive requires the knowledge of an expert familiar with doing so. Careful consideration must be made not to overwhelm the person and their financial situation, and actual needs.

Key Areas To Address For Easing Chronic Pain

It's easy to get overwhelmed at the vast array of therapeutic options available for chronic pain. This is one of the more challenging issues facing the pain sufferer. The good news is, however, we can take a step back and "chunk" the options into larger categories based on what research shows us is successful. Working down into details within each category can always be done if needed.

1. Pain neuroscience education

New research shows the more you know about pain and how it works, the more likely you are to not only make improvements with various therapies, but also experience reduced pain and develop better coping skills. The majority of individuals suffering from chronic pain have not learned from their health care providers what generates their pain. This lack of understanding keeps people searching for structural-mechanical causes of pain, and pursuing therapies that align with those beliefs. The volume of searches online for topics related to specific muscle problems, postural distortions, and other explanations for physical aches and pains such as fascial restriction is staggering. For example, it's a little known fact that generally all tissues in the body heal in a maximum of 6 months. When pain persists past this point, the issue lies within the brain and nervous system, rather than the tissues. This means there are often multiple factors that are contributing to the pain experience beyond structural elements and, if left unaddressed, will likely lead to treatment failure. As discussed previously, having many conflicting diagnoses and subsequent treatment failures leads to staying stuck in the vicious chronic pain cycle. Pain neuroscience education is an established approach designed to educate chronic pain sufferers about their pain to help them move better, exercise with a greater degree of tolerance, experience less suffering, and regain their hope.

2. Sleep

Sleep is essential for life, and every organism with a nervous system requires this type of resting phase. Moreover, it is noted that other types of organisms without a brain do have a circadian rhythm as well. This only highlights the importance of sleep in the physiology of living beings. It is further noted that sleep deprivation is associated with many diseases, including mental health problems, impairment in the immune system, and metabolic dysfunction, including obesity and type 2 diabetes.

The connection between chronic pain and sleep deprivation has been established for a long time. For instance, back in 1979, it was noted in a scientific study that rats that were subjected to sleep deprivation had a significantly lower pain threshold, which means they are more susceptible to pain. More recent studies in humans have confirmed the validity of these findings and that they are a risk factor in people suffering recurrent migraine attacks. Similarly, the current evidence on the matter describes a higher pain perception in various settings, including fibromyalgia, joint dysfunction, and muscle soreness. Not getting enough sleep at night predisposes people to chronic pain and increases the severity of the symptoms and the recurrence of the attacks because it is associated with hyperalgesic changes. In other words, when you don't sleep properly, your body starts feeling pain differently. Besides clinical trials on migraines, there is plenty of supporting evidence to show a definite link between sleep fragmentation or deprivation and chronic pain. We can see the scientific evidence in various medical settings:

- Arthritis and joint pain: According to a clinical trial published in 2016, sleep fragmentation induces an increased sensitization to joint pain. The study compared patients with knee arthritis with a healthy sleep pattern with others who did not sleep properly. After this comparison, the authors concluded that treating sleep is fundamental to improving chronic pain in patients with arthritis.

- Fibromyalgia: This is a condition that features chronic pain, and it is often difficult to trace and diagnose.

- Insomnia is strongly associated with anxiety (not as a result of pain but as an aggravating factor).

- Low back pain: It is a common problem, and most people have at least one episode throughout their lifetime. However, it was found that 53% of people with chronic symptoms of low back pain have sleep problems compared to 3% of pain-free patients who reported insomnia.

- Other musculoskeletal problems: One of the first associations between sleep deprivation and the pain centers on the issue of musculoskeletal symptoms. Sleep-deprived patients report an increase in muscle tenderness and more frequent musculoskeletal symptoms.

- Moreover, recent findings pointed out that the perception of musculoskeletal pain in these patients is increased by 24%.

People who do not sleep properly have a higher sensitivity to pain. According to the evidence published in the journal Psychosomatic Medicine, when pain sensitivity is increased, it is possible to measure this organic change, and there's no additional alteration in perceptions that may contribute to bias. There were no studies on brain perception of pain during periods of sleep deprivation until recently. For instance, healthy young people who do not sleep properly have higher activity in brain areas that trigger pain (the primary somatosensory cortex) and reduced activity in brain areas that coordinate movement and modulate the perception of pain (the insular cortex and the striatum). After the above-mentioned study, practitioners could trace the exact reason why sleep deprivation modulates pain. Sleep deprivation and higher sensitivity to pain increase the sensitivity of the neural network, primarily focusing on neurons that trigger anxiety. At the same time, the body becomes unable to modulate or mute pain sensation and perceives more sharply these sensory impulses. Moreover, the study found that even mild sleep deprivation affects pain perception. Similarly, it should be a wakeup call for anyone who has a continually disrupted sleep pattern and feels any type of pain symptom the day after.

Insomnia hurts, and there's much we can do about it. One of the most severe chronic pain diseases is fibromyalgia, and according to a clinical trial, applying a few sleep hygiene tips has been found to improve the symptoms in these patients. Recommendations include sleeping every day at the same hour; not using the same room to sleep, eat, and study; turning off screens before going to sleep; and avoiding coffee, alcohol, tobacco, and dense, greasy foods. There are many ways to improve our quality of sleep and reduce our perception of chronic pain. What we have to do is raise our awareness of the importance of sleep and follow easy recommendations.

3. Movement

Pain education is critical before engaging in an exercise program. Competent practitioners should possess knowledge about how to set proper expectations and be able to adjust what is being done based on how the patient responds.

When it comes to strength training and chronic pain, the most basic purpose of strength training is to strengthen the larger muscle groups of the body in the basic movement patterns (push, pull, squat, bench, lunge, and twist). These fundamental large muscle groups can, if conditioned, properly help in rehabilitation.

Strength training exercises improve conditioning, build confidence in your ability to do things like bend and lift, and prepare you for physical activities. In time, patients can reduce soreness and strain, enabling them to become less sensitive and more resilient. We call this "building a bigger cup."

Research shows that beginners gain significant benefits from lower resistance, higher repetitions, and a smaller amount of sets. For example, two sets of 20 repetitions of an exercise a few times a week can provide significant benefits. Research shows the benefits of a general exercise prescription vs. individual "core" or postural exercises to be almost identical. However, I find that tailoring exercises specific to the individual's needs is ideal. For example, if someone is afraid to bend forward in fear of making a bulging disc worse, then specific exercises aimed at feeling stronger and more confident at hip hinging are going to work better.

Many people in chronic pain may have difficulty with super-specific "stabilization" exercises for smaller muscles. There is a reason for this. The motor cortex may be utilized in the pain neuro-matrix, thus leaving them decreased importance in excellent motor control. Why?

Because the system is in "threat"! Altered cortisol representation (smudging) may also be involved. If any of this is the case, it's not a problem. Simply allow for a more generalized approach or exercise until things calm down and, if necessary, revisit these movements again later. The level of fitness of the person determines what is "ideal" for that person. A low-intensity exercise (like a 135-lb Romanian deadlift) will be very intense for a person who has never set foot in a gym with chronic lower back pain. (Using a pair of 10-lb dumbbells for a Romanian deadlift would be recommended.) Experienced gym-goers or athletes may not need to regress movement all the way down to isolation exercises to make progress. They may just need modifications to their current exercise program. Beginners will likely need coaching on basic exercises. Squats, deadlifts, pushups, rows, and prerequisites are relatively "isolated" drills to learn proper motor control and awareness of muscles and movements.

A gradual and mentorial approach to training can help reduce the fear of movement and build confidence as long as progressive movement and fitness principles are applied. I like to assign activities based on the opposite pattern identified (movement/posture). If a posture and movement defined are associated with the pain experience, I would address the muscles/actions in the antagonistic pattern. I then assess for differences in pain experience and awareness, depending on the exercise.

What does the research say about movement? There are few things in the health field as versatile as exercise. It is commonly recommended and sometimes prescribed as part of the therapy for various health con-

139

ditions. Even though we assume this type of recommendation for people with excess weight and even cardiovascular issues, it is also beneficial for people that suffer from chronic pain. First, before diving into this topic, we need to separate exercise into two main types: aerobic and anaerobic. Aerobic exercise is also known as cardiovascular (cardio), and anaerobic exercise is known as resistance training, weight training, or strength training. Below, we'll evaluate what the research shows when it comes to the effective use of anaerobic training to relieve chronic pain. Do pain symptoms improve with resistance training?

While many studies show that resistance training generally improves pain symptoms, others show it might not be all that useful. This discrepancy exists because of the type of pain that is being experienced and, of course, the WAY the training is being performed affects a patient's reporting.

If you have a properly designed program, and you're doing everything correctly, you'll be likely to get improvement from some types of chronic pain. A recent analysis of resistance training and chronic lower back pain demonstrates that aerobic exercise and resistance training are both beneficial. A significant reduction of pain intensity was experienced in both groups.

However, resistance exercise displayed an added benefit, the psychological well- being of the individual, which is essential to modulate the perception of pain. It's also interesting to note that there are many variants of resistance training, and each of them has proved to reduce pain in a different way. For instance, we can divide resistance training into static and dynamic muscle contractions. Static muscle contraction, which includes isometric exercise (muscle contraction with no movement), is associated with a moderate-to-large modulation of pain, and specific studies have found that maintaining contraction at a low weight for a longer time recruits and exhausts more muscle fibers, leading to a more significant exercise- induced hypoalgesia. On the other hand, dynamic resistance, which is performed mostly by shortening and lengthening the muscles, has been found to have similar effects, but usually in the short term.

When and how is strength training appropriate for chronic pain? Resistance training can be utilized for various types of chronic pain, including fibromyalgia, which is known to be a reasonably challenging condition. Fibromyalgia is a painful condition that is highly variable between people that have it, and it's associated ultimately with a dysfunction of the nervous system and increased susceptibility to the pain experience. Most of the information out there shows that controlling pain in fibromyalgia is an extremely challenging venture. Even so, "old-school" resistance training is still an effective way to reduce the sensation of pain and tenderness and maintain or increase muscle strength in these individuals.

According to a Cochrane review, aerobic exercise is superior to moderate- intensity resistance training, so it appears to be a good idea to combine them. One of the more common applications of resistance training in chronic pain is associated with things like repetitive strain injuries. For example, a randomized control trial focused on strength training to treat working populations that had repetitive strain injuries, some of which had a work disability. They underwent 10 weeks of strength training against the usual ergonomic care that is recommended to address this kind of pain. Strength training showed significant improvements in hand/wrist pain and reduced time to fatigue by an impressive 97%. Achieving these improvements in chronic pain with resistance exercise is not so difficult. We can choose critical exercises per muscle group, including one or two sets for each exercise. Then select the appropriate weight to perform a correct technique without a problem, and rest between sets for a few minutes. Each repetition should be performed at medium speed, and doing this twice every week for each muscle group is usually enough for good. Current recommendations of physical activity for health by the World Health Organization include 150 minutes of moderate physical activity (aerobic exercise) a week combined with muscle-strengthening activities 2 days a week or more (6).

Common obstacles and risks of resistance training

Generally, to be effective, resistance training needs to be done two to three times per week. This sounds easy, but there are some obstacles to be aware of.

- You may not feel immediate improvements. Even though there's a connection between resistance training and pain sensitivity, it does not produce rapid shifts in pain perception.
- Massage or relaxation training work in tandem with resistance training.
- Real improvements in this area take time: on average, 10 to 12 weeks.
- Change your lifestyle and habits.
- Resistance training requires time commitment and persistence. If you're not committed or cannot stick to it, you aren't likely to get the outcome you are seeking. Resistance training may not be the thing that everyone needs for their type of chronic pain, or it may not fit into their needs at a particular time. Here are a few more things to be aware of:
- Strength-training injuries: Be careful hitting the weights without Nany professional help; no mastery of exercise plan may not only

reduce the benefits but also get you injured. Getting injured in the process of trying to relieve pain is a common issue, and this is why you should seek help from a professional.

- Imprecise exercise protocols for the type of pain: Certain types of chronic pain won't respond well to aggressive resistance training. Some, like NM fibromyalgia, need to be very carefully monitored because the training program may continually need to be adjusted based on how the person is feeling. Frozen shoulder is another issue that may not respond well to strength training at all, and, in fact, it may make it much worse.

Resistance training (anaerobic exercise) certainly has its place in the therapeutic regime of the chronic pain sufferer. It is highly effective, but it must be applied to the right kind of pain issue, in the right way, and progress over time as the person adapts to the program. Exercise is often recommended for many different health conditions, especially those related to the cardiovascular system. Still, it's certainly not the only area where it may be precious. Living a sedentary lifestyle is a fairly significant risk factor for health issues, and it is not only limited to stroke and heart disease. Although many people are apprehensive of being more active when they have pain, studies show that physical activity improves symptoms of chronic pain in the short and long term. There are two primary forms of physical activity (aerobic and anaerobic), and each of them is associated with an improvement in chronic pain.

We're going to focus on aerobic exercise (often referred to as "cardio") and how pain mechanisms can be inhibited by this simple form of movement.

What happens when you do aerobic exercise? During aerobic exercise, the most significant changes involve the respiration and cardiovascular systems. Your muscles play an essential part, and the stroke volume of your heart increases to make up for the increased requirement of oxygen and nutrients. The function of your capillaries is enhanced, and the parts of your cells that produce energy, called mitochondria, increase in both number and efficiency.

Additionally, there are many nervous system and hormonal adaptations that occur after aerobic exercise. These changes improve both strength and stamina and have the ability to reduce insulin resistance and other metabolic problems. Aerobic exercise can also play a role in improving flexibility, balance, and coordination and also positively impact muscle/postural asymmetry. All of these improvements can be associated with various pain inhibitory mechanisms that we discuss below.

How does aerobic exercise inhibit pain? The exact mechanism by which physical activity improves chronic pain symptoms is not entirely understood. Unfortunately, the vast majority of clinical trials do not make a clear distinction between aerobic and anaerobic physical activity when examining the effects of exercise on pain perception. Studies are composed of interventions, therapeutic recommendations, and patient education. The variety of sources makes it challenging to set aside and evaluate the differences between aerobic and anaerobic exercise separately.

A distinction based on short- and long-term effects of aerobic exercise:

Short-term pain inhibition from aerobic exercise

Reduction of pain perception, called hypoalgesia, has been reported after physical activity in healthy individuals, people with chronic pain, and people with experimentally induced pain. The two mechanisms involved in the short-term numbing effect are the release of endorphins and a modulation in the pain pathways in the central nervous system.

According to studies, after high-intensity aerobic exercise, there's a hypoalgesic (numbing) effect lasting approximately 30 minutes. This effect is longer compared to that after resistance-training exercise (anaerobic exercise), which lasts only a few minutes. Studies seem to show that more exercise or higher intensity is related to more hyperalgesia. The suggestion is that to generate a considerable effect, we should engage in high-intensity physical activity for more than 10 minutes or moderate to high physical activity for 30 minutes or more. Now, of course, you can imagine this wouldn't work in many scenarios. For example, some clinical trials have reported an INCREASED pain response instead of pain inhibition in cases of individuals with severe chronic pain. People with fibromyalgia, for example, do not have immediate pain inhibition after physical activity. However, of course, they can still benefit from exercise in the long run.

Long-term pain inhibition from aerobic exercise

The long-term pain inhibitory effects of aerobic exercise are reported only in individuals who maintained a regular program of activity. Long-term activity modulates the endocannabinoid system. These natural cannabis- like molecules produced by the human body reduce inflammation by improving circulation and normalize the transmission of glutamate and pyruvate in the brain and muscle tissue. By altering the release of inflammatory substances and improving circulation, it is possible to reduce swelling and other symptoms that may be associated with some chronic pain issues. Our endocannabinoid system has a strong inhibitory effect that is often targeted by pain medications. The same is also modulated by aerobic activity upon releasing endorphins.

Glutamate and pyruvate are essential for sensory perception in the muscle tissue, the transmission of which is key to the central nervous system. By reducing these substances, physical activity may modulate pain perception in the long run.

The psychological effect of exercise

We can't talk about pain perception without including the cerebral function.

It is well established that depression, anxiety, and similar mental health problems increase pain perception.

Individuals who engage in aerobic exercise usually report a significant improvement in mood and psychological symptoms, which may have a positive effect on the chronic pain experience. There are not, however, enough studies to evaluate these changes in a large number of people suffering from chronic pain.

So, does aerobic exercise help? Yes! In a nutshell, aerobic exercise is known to reduce pain perception immediately after exercise and in the long run. For long- lasting results, it is necessary to engage in sustained activity. In most cases of chronic pain, patients would also benefit from combining some aerobic exercise with anaerobic exercise. By joining the strengthening nature of anaerobic exercise and the physiological changes mentioned in this chapter, it is possible to reduce pain symptoms and improve the quality of life for chronic pain sufferers.

4. Goal setting

Pain relief should not be the only target of a therapeutic program. While obviously an important one, some types of chronic pain conditions do not simply go away completely. Instead, one must learn how to live alongside it. As sensitivity to pain is high already in those with chronic pain, continuing to solely focus on the changes in pain sensitivity by itself often leads to greater frustration, worry, fear, anxiety and therefore more pain.

Improved function on the other hand leads to improvement in quality of life and improved coping. One of the most debilitating aspects of chronic pain is the effect it has on an individual's ability to be active, work, and play. When pain can be reduced, these activities can often be modified and returned to, leading to positive impact on all elements of the biopsychosocial system. This in turn leads to sending more messages of safety to the nervous system, which often results in less pain. For some, the road to where they want to be may be long, which can be overwhelming without setting smaller, attainable goals that inspire, motivate, and reward accomplishments. Dealing with a lot of common life stressors on top of dealing with pain can be very overwhelming. This can sap your energy and wear you down as life's demands stack up. Setting priorities and simple goals to do a little at a time can add up over time and reduce the sensitivity of your alarm system, and therefore pain.

While these are the largest and arguably the most important categories that are needed to address chronic pain, they certainly aren't the only helpful ones. The importance of addressing nutrition, application of manual therapies, and mindfulness techniques such as meditation, hypnotherapy, or even psychological counseling should not be overlooked as important therapeutic interventions to employ.

I hope this chapter has shed some light on how to approach your chronic pain with an updated, scientific rationale, and make educated and informed decisions based on what the current research suggests. Numerous additional areas are currently being studied, such as the role of inflammation and nutritional strategies to reduce sensitivity in chronic pain. These approaches are very promising, with many healthcare providers achieving successful outcomes currently. We anxiously await their findings in order to expand our knowledge and provide even more resources to chronic pain sufferers.

WORKS CITED

Augle, K. M., & Riley 3rd, J. L. (2014). Self-reported physical activity predicts pain inhibitory and facilitatory function. Medicine and science in sports and exercise, 46(3), 622.

Bender, T., Nagy, G., Barna, I., Tefner, I., Kádas, É., & Géher, P. (2007). The effect of physical therapy on beta-endorphin levels. European journal of applied physiology, 100(4), 371-382.

Gerdle, B., Ernberg, M., Mannerkorpi, K., Larsson, B., Kosek, E., Christidis, N., & Ghafouri, B. (2016). Increased interstitial concentrations of glutamate and pyruvate in vastus lateralis of women with fibromyalgia syndrome are normalized after an exercise intervention–a case-control study. PloS one, 11(10), e0162010.

Ghafouri, N., Ghafouri, B., Fowler, C. J., Larsson, B., Turkina, M. V., Karlsson, L., & Gerdle, B. (2014). Effects of two different specific neck exercise interventions on palmitoylethanolamide stearoylethanolamide concentrationsin the interstitium of the trapezius muscle in women with chronic neckshoulder pain. *Pain Medicine*, 15(8), 1379-1389.

Kawi, J., Lukkahatai, N., Inouye, J., Thomason, D., & Connelly, K. (2016). Effects of exercise on select biomarkers and associated outcomes   chronic pain conditions: systematic review. Biological research for nursing, 18(2), 147-159.

Kisner, Colby, Borstad. Title: Therapeutic Exercise: Foundations and Techniques.F.A. Davis Company, 2018.

Koltyn, K. F. (2002). Exercise-induced hypoalgesia and intensity of exercise. Sports medicine, 32(8), 477-487.

Liebenson,. Craig, Rehabilitation of the Spine : a Practitioner's Manual. Philadelphia :Lippincott Williams & Wilkins, 2003.

Morris, Craig. Title: Low Back Syndromes: Integrated Clinical. McGraw-Hill Medical/Jaypee Brothers Medical Publishers, 2005.

Naugle, K. M., Fillingim, R. B., & Riley III, J. L. (2012). A meta- analytic review of the hypoalgesic effects of exercise. The Journal of pain, 13(12), 1139-1150.

Nijs, J., Kosek, E., Van Oosterwijck, J., & Meeus, M. (2012). Dysfunctional endogenous analgesia during exercise in patients with chronic pain: to exercise or not to exercise?. Pain physician, 15(3S), ES205-ES213.

Occupational Hearing Loss · Workers Compensation. https:// www.napolilaw. com/practice-areas/workers-compensation/ occupational-hearing-loss/

Sajedi, H., & Bas, M. (2016). The evaluation of the aerobic exercise effects on pain tolerance. Sport Science, 9, 7-11.

Visnic, Sam. Why Didn't My Doctor Tell Me That? 2020. Visnic Center For Integrated Health Inc. and Sam Visnic.

https://content.iospress.com/articles/journal-of-back-andmusculoskeletal- rehabilitation/bmr170920

https://www.sciencedirect.com/science/article/abs/pii/S1526590012008085

https://www.cochranelibrary.com/cdsr/doi/10.1002/14651858. CD010884/ abstract

https://www.hindawi.com/journals/bmri/2016/4137918/abs/

https://www.ncbi.nlm.nih.gov/books/NBK305057/

CHAPTER VII

Sleep, Nutrition, Stress Management
Dr. Lanae Mullane

Welcome to my chapter discussing the biopsychosocial aspects of the foundations of health with a focus on stress management, restorative sleep, and balanced nutrition. My name is Dr. Lanae Mullane, a naturopathic doctor (ND) practicing in California. I completed my training at Bastyr University, nestled in the beautiful Saint Edward State Park in Kenmore, Washington. After graduating, I was just the second ND to complete a residency alongside a rheumatologist.

My philosophy of medicine is rooted in the idea that it takes a village to treat a patient and that each healthcare provider plays a vital role in that patient's outcome and healthcare journey. Throughout my residency and career history, I have chosen to work within integrative health clinics with medical doctors, doctors of osteopathic medicine, and registered dieticians. Providing care in these settings allows for the strengths of each form of medicine to shine through to give a genuinely whole- person approach to treating patients.

Currently, I work as the Director of Nutrition for Vejo. Our company uses a portable, pod-based blender utilizing farm-fresh freeze-dried fruit and vegetable biodegradable blends in formulas to help people live happier and healthier lives. I am also the medical director of a wellness-based clinic called Vejo+ that focuses on optimizing health with evidence-based treatments through laboratory testing, nutraceutical recommendations, and personalized lifestyle and behavioral changes. All Vejo+ members start with an in-depth look at their fundamentals of health because creating a solid foundation is vital in developing resilience.

What is Naturopathic Medicine?

Naturopathic medicine is a distinct healthcare profession rooted in the wisdom of nature that still follows modern scientific standards of care. Naturopathic doctors are trained in rigorous doctoral-level medical education at one of seven accredited naturopathic medical school programs in North America. NDs use evidence- informed therapies focusing on an individualized, whole-person approach to support the body's innate ability to heal while working to identify the root cause of illness. The basis of the practice of naturopathic medicine is established in the six naturopathic principles.

The Six Naturopathic Principles:

1. First, Do No Harm (Primum non nocere): Choosing the least invasive and least toxic therapies, referring to an appropriate provider when a patient's presentation is outside of scope.

2. The Healing Power of Nature (Vis medicatrix naturae): Creating a healthy environment as the foundation to human health by utilizing substances that originate in nature to support the body's innate wisdom to heal itself.

3. Identify and Treat the Causes (Tolle causam): Identifying, addressing, and removing the underlying cause of illness.

4. Doctor as Teacher (Docere): Supporting and empowering patients in their health management through education.

5. Treat the Whole Person (Tolle totum): Treating the patient, not the disease, by identifying the interconnectedness of our body to our environment and lifestyle as an integrated whole of total health.

6. Prevention (Praevenic): Focusing on overall wellness and disease prevention utilizing these six principles to identify potential areas of imbalance to educate patients on how to get and stay well.

A common misconception is that NDs are homeopaths. Homeopathy is the treatment of ailments using minute doses of natural substances that in a healthy person would produce symptoms of the disease. While NDs have some training in the modality of homeopathy, not all NDs use it in their practice. NDs are united more by the dynamic philosophy of the Naturopathic Principles and Therapeutic Order than a specific modality of medicine. Naturopathic treatments can include botanical medicine, nutrition, hydrotherapy, pharmaceuticals, minor surgery, and lifestyle and behavioral changes.

Building Resilience Through the Fundamentals of Health

Creating the foundation for one's health has always been a staple in naturopathic philosophy. Considering recent world events, paying attention to wellness has become even more vital. Building resilience through focusing on the fundamentals helps our body withstand, adapt to, and recover quickly from adversity and unfavorable situations that challenge our health. Some may be born resilient, but our bodies can also improve our innate resilience. Concerning health, this idea can be achieved by optimizing three critical aspects of wellness: stress management, restorative sleep, and balanced nutrition. By focusing on the fundamentals, we create healthy soil for our bodies to flourish and thrive I will be breaking down the three aspects of foundational wellness by discussing the biology, psychosocial, and contextual features of naturopathy alongside integrative approaches that can influence one's health resilience.

Stress Management

Biological: How stress affects our body

The stress response is a standard and adaptive coping mechanism that humans have relied on for millions of years for protection (e.g., running from a bear in the wild). The stress response was designed exceptionally well for acute stressors that resolve quickly. Unfortunately, in our modern society, daily life events can lead to chronic or continuous mild stress exposures. The physiological stress response—higher heart rate, shallow and rapid breathing, increased release of adrenaline, noradrenaline, and cortisol—can occur whether you are running from a bear or sitting in the morning rush hour. As complex as the body is, it is not necessarily able to discern the differences between stressors.

Within the body, the neuroendocrine adaptation component of the stress response system is known as the hypothalamic-pituitary-adrenal axis (HPA axis). Once the body perceives the presence of a stressor, a cascade of biological events occurs, starting in an area of the brain called the hypothalamus. The hypothalamus maintains homeostasis by responding to various signals from the internal and external environment, including hunger, blood pressure, thermoregulation, and hormones. The hypothalamus releases corticotropin-releasing hormone (CRH) to the pituitary gland, sending a message via adrenocorticotropic hormone (ACTH) through the blood to the adrenal glands, which sit on top of both kidneys. The adrenal glands secrete cortisol, the "stress hormone," which controls a vast array of physiological processes, such as metabolic (raising blood sugar), immune (weakening immune response), ion transport (preventing sodium loss and accelerating potassium excretion from a cell), and memory (overwhelming the hippocampus, causing atrophy). The circulating cortisol activates a "negative feedback loop" in which the hypothalamus ceases production of

CRH, which stops the pituitary from creating ACTH, thus returning the body to homeostasis.

You may also feel the physiologic effects of stress in the gastrointestinal tract: Have you ever had a "gut feeling"? That has to do with the gut-brain axis. The gut is sometimes called the "second brain" or the enteric nervous system, consisting of millions of nerve cells that line the gastrointestinal tract from the mouth to the rectum. The brain has direct effects on the digestive tract, including the stomach and intestines. The mere thought of eating food can release digestive enzymes in saliva, the stomach, and the pancreas before you even place a bite in your mouth. Issues in the gut can send signals to the brain, just as issues in the brain can signal the digestive tract; the gut and the brain are closely interconnected: Are digestive issues the cause or the result of stress and anxiety? What's more, the lining of the digestive tract also contains a majority of your body's serotonin receptors, and serotonin is a chemical needed for nerve cells and brain function and also plays a critical role in mood and cognition.

In addition to cortisol and gastrointestinal health, prolonged exposure to chronic stress can have negative impacts on numerous other areas of health, including disrupting the digestive, immune, sleep, reproductive, and cardiovascular systems and leading to heart disease, weight changes, high blood pressure, anxiety, depression, and diabetes.

Psychosocial: Daily adverse experiences and our ability to cope

The impacts of stress and adversity can be physiological, as noted above, and psychological, affecting people's social behavior. Stress can have a powerful influence on one's ability to show empathy and financial generosity, and can promote aggressive behavior or perpetuate violence. Exposures to stress as early as pre-conception, prenatal, or infancy can contribute to variable health outcomes, from chronic metabolic diseases to developmental delays. Adverse childhood experiences (ACEs) have been shown to create excessive activation of the stress response, leading to long-term mental and physical repercussions. Research is now trying to understand better how experiences transmitted through generational trauma can alter DNA (called cross-generational epigenetics).

Since 2007, the American Psychological Association (APA) has issued a yearly survey, Stress in AmericaTM, to people in the United States to identify the leading causes and impacts of stress. Throughout the thirteen surveys conducted, the contributors of external stress were influenced by economic decline, political conflict, racial disparities, and discrimination. The impact of the COVID pandemic highlighted increased stress in 2020. Most adults in the U.S. report experiencing daily discrimination based on age, race, disability, gender, sexual orientation, and gender identity.1 The results of these discriminations can lead to heightened vigilance and changes in behavior, which can initiate the stress cascade contributing to poorer health outcomes.

Contextual: Impact of environment on stress

Our environment can have a profound impact on both physiological and psychosocial contributions to stress. Commuting in Los Angeles for years, I can personally acknowledge the increase in blood pressure and shortness of breath when sitting in bumper-to-bumper traffic. Having also lived in Seattle for school, I have experienced the lack of sun and its influence on the seasonal affective disorder. Our surroundings—whether loud noises, lack of personal space, food unavailability, or chemical exposures—affect our daily stress response.

Exposures to environmental toxins can also act as facilitators of chronic disease. We are likely exposed to hundreds of these daily without even realizing it. This exposure contributes to physiologic stress in the body (and the planet). Environmental toxins are also referred to as endocrine- disrupting chemicals (EDC) or hormone-disrupting chemicals. EDCs are external chemicals that interfere with any aspect of hormonal action and have been found in breast milk, blood, and urine. The endocrine system includes glands and receptors in tissues and organs that respond to hormones. Small exposures over time accumulate to measurable levels in the human body. They can contribute to adverse health outcomes like cancer, reproductive complications, and cardiovascular and metabolic diseases through oxidative stress, autonomic imbalance, vascular dysfunction, systemic inflammation, and HPA activation.

Some of the more notorious environmental toxins that people are exposed to are:

- Glyphosates are found in weed killers.
- Polychlorinated biphenyls (PCBs) are found in oil-based paint, insulation, electrical equipment, and caulking material.
- Bisphenol A (BPA) is found in hard/rigid plastics, metal food cans, thermal receipts.
- Phthalates are found in toys, detergents, lubricating oils, food packaging, pharmaceuticals, and vinyl floors.
- Parabens are antimicrobial preservatives found in personal care products.

Stress Management: An integrative approach to stress

No one is immune to stress; however, it is possible to change our body's response to it. The process may not be easy and will likely take some practice, yet one of the fastest, most cost-effective stress-reducing techniques is utilizing the power of the breath. Breathing is controlled by the autonomic nervous system, which allows a person to continue to breathe while sleeping or unconscious; it simultaneously will enable one to control the rate of breath consciously. Although breathing is something people have been doing since birth, we are not always the most efficient. Poor posture, shallow breathing, and breath-holding are common occurrences that we are conditioned to in our busy lives and our more sedentary computer work environments. Conscious breathing is an essential step in the reduction of stress.

Supporting an optimal breathing environment begins before the inhale. Start with your feet flat on the floor with the body in an upright position and shoulders relaxed. To remove "accessory" muscles that contribute to more shallow chest breathing, place hands on both sides near the lowest ribs. Inhale through the nose, pause, and exhale through the mouth. Allow the exhale to be longer than the inhale, as the exhale stimulates the parasympathetic nervous system via stimulation of the vagus nerve on the diaphragm, telling the brain to relax. When doing breathing exercises, to reduce the risk of feeling light-headed, place more emphasis on the rate of the breath versus the volume. Pursing the lips as if drinking through a straw when exhaling can help slow down the rate. Repeat at least four times. Once behavioral tools are in place, a medical professional may want to do salivary cortisol testing, followed by herbal nutraceuticals to support cortisol homeostasis. A form of nutraceutical, adaptogens have been used for centuries worldwide to modulate cortisol balance by structurally resembling adrenal hormones.

Some of the more commonly used adaptogenic herbs are ashwagandha (Withania somnifera), astragalus (Astragalus membranaceus), Rhodiola (Rhodiola rosea), and eleuthero (Eleutherococcus senticosus).

Another way to reduce environmental stress is to limit exposure to EDCs in toxic chemicals. Avoid plastics with recycling #3 and #7, food wrapped in plastic packaging, heating food in plastic containers, and canned foods. When possible, consume foods that are fresh, frozen, or organic. Use glass or stainless steel containers and hand-wash plastic containers. Go paperless and say no to thermal receipts. Cleanse your home and body with natural cleaning products. For more helpful resources, the Environmental Working Group has created a repository of products rated from least to most toxic.

Chronic stress comes in many shapes and forms, from physiological to emotional to environmental, all carrying potential negative health implications. Your ability to control some stressors may be unlikely, but your ability to control how your body responds to that stress is more likely. As a society, acknowledging the detrimental impacts of stress by supporting healthier work environments/requirements, dismantling racial disparities, providing access to healthcare, creating more inclusive spaces, reducing environmental toxins, and offering more mental health support would help minimize exposure to stressors. On an individual level, try to incorporate stress management techniques into your daily routine to increase the usefulness of your tools; this way, you can combat stressors as they arise. Find a stress management technique that works for you, whether that is breathing techniques, movement, talking to friends, utilizing the expertise of a therapist, being out in nature, or scheduling a bi-monthly massage. Whatever you choose, strive to make it a ritual in your self-care practice.

Sleep

Biological: How sleep affects our body

Sleep is one of the most important components to establishing a foundation of health. An inability to achieve restorative sleep leads to profound stress in the body, contributing to poor health outcomes such as chronic illness, mood disorders, hormone dysregulation, immune dysfunction, and insulin resistance. In children and young adults, sleep is when the human growth hormone is released to help with development. Sleep helps create new synapses in the brain. And yet, a growing number of people battle with nonrestorative sleep or sleep that does not result in a feeling of being rested. Research for optimal quantities of hours of sleep for overall health is still being developed. Still, the current consensus for an adult is seven to nine hours, with younger populations needing more. Lack of sleep is known to affect memory, performance, and lifespan negatively. A CDC survey reported that adults who received less than the recommended seven hours of sleep were more likely to report ten chronic health conditions, including depression, arthritis, and diabetes.[2]

To reach restorative sleep, we need to address both sleep quality and quantity. Sleep quality refers to uninterrupted sleep that reaches each stage of the sleep cycle: awake, light sleep, deep sleep, and REM sleep. These stages may also be referred to as NREM (non-rapid eye movement) and REM (rapid eye movement). Generally, the body will transition through each cycle stage sequentially four to five times over 90 minutes, with earlier sleep tending to favor deep sleep, while later in the night selecting more REM sleep.

Sleep itself plays a vital role in the regulation of hormones. As the sun sets and the light dims, your body naturally produces the hormone melatonin. Melatonin does not make you sleep but does contribute to a sensation of heavy eyelids and quiet wakefulness that prepares the body for sleep. Jet lag, change in time zones, or working night shifts can impact the body's melatonin production. Sleep is also crucial for regulating cortisol and testosterone; poor sleep quality or insufficient sleep can disrupt endocrine production. As discussed previously, cortisol is the body's stress hormone produced by the adrenal glands. Disruption of cortisol can lead to issues with the digestive, immune, sleep, reproductive, and cardiovascular systems. In cisgender men, most testosterone is released during sleep, and sleep deprivation is associated with producing lower amounts of testosterone, essential for reproduction, libido, muscle mass, and bone density.

In menstruating females, menstrual cycles have been linked to disruptions in circadian rhythms with reported inferior sleep quality during the premenstrual week. Women in the perimenopausal stage are the most likely to struggle with insomnia.

The sleep-immune connection is clear: There is no doubt that an illness can lead to an increased feeling of being tired, and a good night's sleep is commonly recommended when feeling under the weather. Sleep influences the immune system through proteins called cytokines, which not only support a restful night's sleep but also increase when there is an infection or inflammation. A lack of sleep can lower the body's production of these cytokines and weaken the body's defense system. This response can increase susceptibility to cold and flu infections, as well as affect how fast someone may recover once sick.

Psychosocial: Societal influences on sleep behavior

While diagnosable sleep disorders such as insomnia, narcolepsy, sleep apnea, and restless leg syndrome are sleep disruptors, they are not the only contributors to poor sleep. Numerous societal norms contribute to an unrestful night's sleep. Alcohol, caffeine, and sleep medications are some of the top culprits in today's society.

Alcohol is often used to help people unwind from a long day, celebrate the end of a workday, or mitigate stressful life situations due to its sedative effects that can induce a sense of relaxation. A couple of glasses of alcohol may cause a feeling of relaxation, but as the alcohol metabolizes, the relaxing effect wears off. This response disrupts the deep sleep and REM sleep cycles, leading to sleep that is not deep or long in duration; this contributes to extensive adverse effects and increases daytime sleepiness.

Caffeine can trigger our sympathetic "flight, fight, or freeze" response, leading to an increase in epinephrine, also known as adrenaline. This response is the same autonomic nervous system response that our body perceives a situation as problematic or dangerous. Caffeine can cause an increase in heart rate, disruption in sleep, digestive disturbance, irritability, and agitation, all of which can increase your level of perceived stress and anxiety. Genetics may also play a role in how well the body handles caffeine. Variations in the CYP1A2 gene can determine if someone is a fast or slow metabolizer of caffeine. Slow metabolizers take longer for their bodies to process caffeine, contributing to possible adverse effects like insomnia and anxiety. Caffeine is classified as a stimulant drug with the exact mechanism of action as an adenosine receptor antagonist. Adenosine is a somnogenic substance, so caffeine consumption blocks the adenosine receptor, decreasing the sensation of sleepiness.

Medications prescribed or sold over-the-counter for sleep are a blanket approach and do not necessarily address personalized causes of sleep disruption. Current sleeping pills do not allow for standard patterns of restorative sleep, and most sleeping pills have a mechanism of action that focuses on GABA receptors of the brain to slow down the nervous system. Although these pills can allow a person to fall asleep, inducing a sensation of drowsiness, they can inhibit deeper brain waves during REM sleep, which is beneficial for problem-solving, learning, and memory. Disruptions in the REM sleep cycle may lead to grogginess the following morning. Overlooking the root cause of the sleep disruption can lead to an unhealthy dependence on sleeping pills.

Contextual: Impact of the environment on sleep

The use of portable electronic devices has been normalized in today's society, and it has become commonplace to have a screen in the bedroom. The increase in screen time has contributed to increased non-restorative sleep in children, adolescents, and adults. Screen entertainment can disrupt sleep causing a delay in bedtime, and therefore, shortened sleep duration. The type of media watched before bed, like stimulating video games, news stories, television shows, movies, and social media, have been shown to increase arousal before bed. This is linked to delayed bedtime, an increased heart rate, and disruption to the REM sleep cycle. Similarly, light exposure from screens when the sun goes down has negatively impacted sleep quality and quantity. The evening light exposure maximizes a state of alertness, delaying the onset of sleep while also showing other side effects, such as postponing melatonin production and disrupting the circadian clock and REM sleep cycle.[3]

Shift work schedules, increasingly high-pressure job requirements, and a socioeconomic environment that increases the need for multiple jobs have also been shown to affect sleep negatively. Numerous workers' schedules do not fit into the traditional nine-to-five workday. Many are subject to rotating, longer hours, night, or on-call demands, leading to a disturbance in the natural circadian rhythm. Circadian refers to a cycle of roughly 24 hours that helps the body regulate essential systemic functions, including hunger, hormone levels, body temperature, alertness, and sleepiness. This "internal clock" is influenced by exposure to sunlight, creating a sense of day vs. night cycle. Shift workers have to go against this natural rhythm to stay awake, possibly leading to a loss of hours of sleep within 24 hours, contributing to the adverse effects of sleep deviation and an increased risk of insomnia.

Achieving Restorative Sleep: An integrative approach to sleep

As fundamental as sleep is to overall health, achieving restorative sleep can be challenging. When working with patients with disordered sleep, after ruling out pathology, the first area we address is called sleep hygiene. These are the different practices or rituals that support an environment for restorative night sleep, as well as full daytime alertness. This starts with keeping the bedroom for sleep and intimacy only as removing distractions allow your mind to acknowledge that your bed is a place for rest. Setting the thermostat cooler around 60-67o F can help make it easier to fall and stay asleep.

Setting a consistent bedtime is also important. As complex as the human body is, when it comes to sleep, the body prefers to keep it simple with routine. Maintaining a regular sleep-wake schedule (which includes weekdays and weekends), the body will support the internal clock by making it easier to fall asleep and wake up. Another important sleep hygiene tip is to turn off or set aside all electronic media devices about an hour before bed to calm the nervous system and reduce blue light exposures that can lower the body's production of melatonin.

If falling asleep is difficult, progressive muscle relaxation, or PMR, may be helpful. This distraction technique was introduced in the 1930s by a physician named Edmund Jacobson and involved rotating between contraction and relaxation of major muscle groups throughout the body. There are numerous ways to practice PMR, and here is an example that patients have found successful. The body should be situated in a comfortable position in a quiet environment. Starting with the toes, contract by curling the toes, then slowly release, counting to 30 seconds. Repeat three times. Move to the feet by flexing and slowly relaxing over 30 seconds. Repeat three times. Continue up the calves to the thighs to the glutes, to the hands, arms, neck, shoulders, jaw, and forehead. If a wandering thought enters your mind, start back at the toes. Most find it difficult to get past the thighs before falling asleep.

For some, falling asleep is the easy part, but staying asleep is more complicated. If awakened during the night and unable to fall asleep after roughly 15 minutes, get out of bed. The bed should only be used for sleep and intimacy. Tossing and turning for long periods can lead to an increased sensation of anxiety. The recommendation is to get out of bed and sit in a chair, listen to soft music, or turn on low light to read until you feel drowsy, then go back to bed. A possible culprit causing people to wake during the night may be a dip in blood sugar levels. This dip does not necessarily need to be large enough to be considered a hypoglycemic event but is enough to alert the body to wake. This is more common in people who eat dinner early—consuming a small handful of healthy fat or protein, like nuts, 30 minutes to an hour before bed can be enough to stabilize the blood sugar and keep a person asleep.

As I noted, caffeine is classified as a stimulant substance that can contribute to difficulty falling asleep. However, the FDA considers

400mg of caffeine (three to four cups of coffee) per day to be safe, limiting caffeine intake to no more than one to two cups of coffee before noon can make sleeping easier. For some, switching to a lower caffeine drink such as matcha or green tea or eliminating caffeine ultimately may be necessary.

Herbs can be a gentle approach to add to your sleep routine. Herbal teas with nervine botanicals promote relaxation for natural sleep. They include chamomile (Matricaria chamomilla), hops (Humulus lupulus), lavender (Lavendula Officinalis), lemon balm (Melissa officinalis), passionflower (Passiflora incarnata), skullcap (Scutellaria laterifolia), and valerian (Valeriana officinalis). The ritual of preparing and sipping on warm herbal tea can also be a relaxing addition to one's sleep hygiene routine. To avoid waking to urinate at night, have a cup or two an hour before bed.

Nutraceuticals may be needed as a slightly higher intervention than behavioral changes for the treatment of poor sleep. Magnesium is involved in over 300 different biochemical reactions in the body, including acting as a natural antagonist of N-Methyl-D-aspartic acid (NMDA) and an agonist of Gamma-aminobutyric acid (GABA), as well as playing a role in the regulation of central nervous system excitability, all of which are important in sleep regulation. Although magnesium is found in nuts, seeds, whole grains, and leafy greens, diets higher in more processed foods and soil nutrient depletion may be contributing to increased cases of magnesium deficiency. Plus, the form of magnesium matters. Cheaper forms of magnesium, like magnesium oxide, are poorly absorbed, contributing to a more laxative effect. The recommended form of magnesium for sleep is magnesium glycinate (a chelate of magnesium with the amino acid glycine). This is a bioavailable form that has been shown to improve sleep quality.

Other favorable supplements used to support sleep include 5-HTP, GABA, and melatonin. Serotonin is a precursor of the hormone melatonin and has been implicated in the regulation of sleep. 5-Hydroxytryptophan (5-HTP) is an intermediate metabolite of the essential amino acid L-tryptophan in the production of serotonin. Short-term, oral supplementing with 5-HTP is well absorbed and bypasses the conversion of L-tryptophan into 5-HTP with the aid of tryptophan hydroxylase enzyme. 5-HTP is contraindicated when taking SSRI antidepressants and MAO inhibitors which increase serotonin levels. Gamma-aminobutyric acid (GABA) is an amino acid and inhibitory neurotransmitter. The natural form of GABA can lower stress-related beta waves and increase alpha waves in the brain to create a sensation of physical relaxation and enhanced sleep.

The most popular sleep supplement is melatonin, most commonly used for jet lag, shift work, and primary sleep disorders. The typical dosage of melatonin ranges from 1 mg to 5 mg. A meta-analysis showed that melatonin improved sleep by reducing sleep-onset latency, improving sleep quality, and increasing total sleep time compared to placebo.[4] In contrast to hypnotic sleep medications, the study also found no indications of the development of tolerance with the use of melatonin.[4] Nearly a third of our life is spent sleeping, making sleep one of the body's most important foundations of health. Creating a relaxing environment conducive for the body and mind for sleep, removing potential stimulus triggers during the day, and being consistent with a routine will help set you up for a successful, refreshing night's sleep that supports the immune system, hormones, memory, energy, and overall wellness.

Nutrition

Biological: How nutrition affects the body

When discussing the importance of nutrition and food on our foundation of health, it is essential to understand the relationship between how food is digested and how nutrients are utilized in the body. The terms "gut," digestive tract, or gastrointestinal system refers to the hollow organs of the mouth, esophagus, stomach, small intestine, large intestine, and anus. Although these hollow organs are found inside the body, they are considered "outside" since ingested contents need to be absorbed "inside" the body. If they are not interested, the contents will be excreted. The gastrointestinal system also includes the solid organs of the pancreas, liver, and gallbladder.

In the digestive tract is a complex ecosystem called the microbiome. There are trillions of microorganisms made up of mainly anaerobic (existing in the absence of oxygen) bacteria and fungi, viruses, and parasites. Over 1000 different microbial bacteria species have been identified to reside in the intestinal microbiome.[5] The microbiome starts with exposure to microorganisms as a baby leaves the birth canal and with the introduction of breast milk. Environmental, medication, genetics, and dietary exposures throughout life will alter the microbiome to support health or increase the risk of disease. The microbiota contributes to digestion by synthesizing vitamins and amino acids, communicating with the intestinal cells, and strengthening the immune system. The fluctuating microbiome can be influenced by a diversified diet, adequate dietary fiber, or consumption of processed foods.

In addition to altering our microbiota, food is vital as a foundation for our overall health. The focus on the impact of food on health and disease prevention has always fostered an interest. Over 2000 years ago, Hippocrates espoused us to "Let food be thy medicine and medicine be thy food." A diet depleted of certain nutrients or with an excess of sodium has been linked to increased high blood pressure, cholesterol, type 2 diabetes, certain cancers, and deficits in brain development.

"Functional foods" have risen in popularity recently, and they go beyond providing basic nutrition. They contain potentially positive health benefits and are correlated with a reduction in disease risk. The most commonly used example of functional food is oats. The FDA approved the cholesterol-lowering health claim that oats can reduce the risk of coronary artery disease due to the beta-glucan soluble fiber.

Nutrition impacts each of the body's systems, with nutrition and the endocrine system particularly intricately intertwined. In addition to the endocrine system's role in growth, blood pressure, sleep, and reproduction, this organ system also regulates appetite, metabolism, and nutrient storage, absorption, and use. A protein deficiency can affect the release of gonadal hormones preventing reproduction, low body fat in cisgender females can stop menstruation, and malnourished children produce less growth hormone. Probably the most famous connection between nutrition and the endocrine system is the link between over nutrition of quickly absorbed sugars and empty calories to the development of type 2 diabetes. The body produces insulin from the pancreas to maintain balanced blood sugar, but increased demands for more insulin to keep the blood sugar balanced can eventually lead to insulin resistance, diabetes, and metabolic health problems.

Food quality and quantity are known factors to affect health, but an emerging area of research is exploring the importance of a person's genetic makeup. Nutrigenomics, a portmanteau of nutritional genomics, is an area of science that looks at how food affects our genes. This focus of study aids in the personalization of medicine and health by examining how an individual's genetic makeup affects the body's response to nutrients or bioactive compounds found in the food that they consume. Nutrigenomic research has shown some promising information on biomarkers of metabolic syndrome, nutrient intake, and genetic polymorphisms concerning micronutrient metabolism and absorption. The use of nutrigenomics in a clinical setting to provide applicable, reliable, and predictable dietary recommendations for improved health is still in the early stages of nutrition research, but the potential is exciting.

Psychosocial: Mental health and its influence on nutrition

Mental health should be addressed in a whole-person approach, with nutrition being only one aspect utilized as an adjunctive treatment. As mentioned when discussing the psychosocial element of stress, the enteric nervous system—the gut-brain axis—can influence mood as the gut and the brain are closely connected. The brain has direct effects on the digestive tract, including on the stomach and intestines.

Most bacteria in the digestive tract can produce the neurotransmitters dopamine and serotonin sent to receptors in the brain to influence mood and behavior. While it is important to note that dietary changes alone may not necessarily cure mental health conditions, changes in dietary patterns may help reduce symptoms, increase energy, and support our ability to adapt better to the stress that may contribute to anxiety or depression.

One such diet, the Mediterranean Diet, has been associated with lower cardiovascular risk, and research has shown positive results in this diet's reducing depression- and anxiety-related symptoms. The PREDI-DEP study showed evidence for the effectiveness of using the Mediterranean Diet to prevent the recurrence of depression and improving the quality of life in patients with past reported episodes of depression.[6]The

Mediterranean Diet is based on the eating habits of the traditional cuisine of countries bordering the Mediterranean Sea and consists of a high intake of vegetables, fruits, whole grains, beans, nuts, seeds, and olive oil. The diet recommends choosing poultry and fish over less lean protein sources like red meat, and healthy fats over saturated and trans fats.

The Gut-and-Psychology Syndrome (GAPS) Diet addresses the gutbrain connection, utilizing a dietary plan derived from the Specific Carbohydrate Diet. This dietary plan was created for those suffering from intestinal and neurological conditions due to an imbalance of the microbiota in the digestive tract. GAPS aims to remove foods that can be challenging for the body to digest and may cause disruption to the gut bacteria and replace them with nutrient-dense food options to support a healthy intestinal permeability. This diet can be difficult, and proponents recommended users get support from a doctor or nutritionist trained in GAPS diet protocol.

Specific foods and drinks have been associated with contributing to worsening anxiety and depression. Caffeine can cause an increase in heart rate, disruption in sleep, digestive disturbance, irritability, and agitation; all can increase one's level of perceived stress and anxiety. Alcohol is often used to mitigate stressful life situations due to its sedative-like effects that can cause a sense of relaxation. Although alcohol may reduce anxiety temporarily, it also has the possibility of increasing anxiety within a few hours after consumption that can last into the following day. After the euphoric effects of alcohol fade, the levels of the neurotransmitter serotonin also decrease. This can lead to feelings of anxiousness and depression. Indulging in sugary comfort foods—whether to cope with painful emotions or stress—has been shown to temporarily reduce the activity of our stress response through the HPA axis. Yet, this temporary alleviation of stress can lead to perpetuating emotional eating habits. Consuming sugary foods can also lead to a spike and quick drop in blood sugar that can cause uneasiness, changes in mood, and feelings similar to a panic attack. This can turn into a cycle of gravitating to something sweet every time you need a boost in mood or energy, leading to a rollercoaster of highs and lows that can contribute to anxiety.

Contextual: Impact of environment on what we eat

The environment plays a significant role in the quality and quantity of nutrients found in our food. The use of monoculture agriculture, a single crop in a specific area, negatively impacts our food and environmental ecological systems. Monoculture goes against nature by cultivating a lack of diversity: removing plant species that would provide nutrients to the soil leads to fewer microorganisms and fewer insect species, leading to the possibility that a single population could overwhelm the crops. This then leads to the increased use of synthetic herbicides, insecticides, and fertilizers. Microorganisms cannot process the inorganic material into organic matter, leading to poisons leaching into the soil and potentially polluting groundwater.

Likewise, ease of access to a variety of nutrient-rich foods is a significant public health issue. The USDA's Economic Research Service identified 6,500 food deserts in the United states.[7] Food deserts are areas where the population has limited access to a variety of healthy and affordable food. Locations with a higher percentage of minority populations and higher poverty rates are more likely to experience food deserts. These areas also tend to have limited access to health care, transportation, and recreational areas.

Cultural influences on food choices are commonly overlooked. The Mediterranean and even vegetarian diets have been heavily researched but have left numerous other ethnically diverse diets, such as Native American, African, and Persian. Nutrition experts are looking to change the dialogue. Dr. Kera Nyemb-Diop, who holds a Ph.D. in nutrition science and a master's in food science, works with black women to "decolonize your plate" to nurture the body and let go of food guilt and shame. She believes that food fuels not only the body but also one's heritage and traditions. She sheds light on the lack of research on culturally diverse diets and the trend of labeling traditional black food as "unhealthy."

Balanced Nutrition: An integrative approach to food

Approaching patients with personalized dietary modification interventions has been the most effective way to alter behavior, contributing to long-term success and improved health outcomes. Considering cultural background, medical history, daily output, economic access, relationship to food, goals, dietary sensitivities, and preferences means that a universal dietary recommendation is unlikely to yield sustainable results. Although working with a trained healthcare provider is recommended for guidance and support, individuals can make changes independently.

For those not struggling with specific gastrointestinal complaints but desiring a better understanding of simple changes for nutrition guidance, the Healthy Eating Plate recommendations provided by Harvard's School of Public Health is a good starting point.[8] The Healthy Eating Plate focuses on what's on your plate. One half should consist of assorted colorful vegetables and some fruit, one-fourth of whole grains (e.g., quinoa, brown rice, oats, barley, and whole wheat), one-fourth of protein (e.g., beans, nuts, and fish and poultry; limiting red meat and no processed meats), healthy fats in moderation (olive oil, ghee, coconut oil, avocado, nuts, and seeds), and finishing the plate with water, tea, or coffee. If tolerated, dairy consumption is limited to, at most, two servings daily. The main point is to create a balanced plate with quality ingredients. The use of spices and herbs is not indicated in the recommendations but is encouraged.

For those with gastrointestinal complaints (e.g., bloating, diarrhea, constipation, and gas), skin disorders, fatigue, allergies, and autoimmune conditions where an underlying condition has been diagnosed or ruled out, the Elimination/Re- challenge Program may be recommended. The Elimination/Re-challenge Program is used to identify possible underlying foods contributing to a patient's unwanted symptoms. This is the gold standard for identifying food sensitivities. To begin the Elimination part of the program, an individual removes the most common dietary allergies: dairy, gluten, eggs, soy, nuts, peanuts, shellfish, corn, alcohol, and caffeine for 21 days. The symptom(s) should show an improvement within that time. In specific scenarios, it may be necessary to remove a broader range of foods, including nightshades, legumes, citrus foods, or food colorings. Once the 21 days have been completed, the patient moves from the Elimination phase to the Re-challenge stage, in which a single food group is re-introduced every three days with two to three servings of that particular food item per day. After the three days, the patient will return to the Elimination phase for two days to ensure no delayed sensitivity reactions. If a person does not react, they can move onto the next food group, repeating the process until each food group has been re-introduced. If a patient notices an increase in symptoms when consuming a food group, they should document it and remove that food group from their diet for some time. It is important to note that foods that are identified to contribute to a reaction may be restricted for some time but should be re-challenged once gut health is addressed. For identifying possible life-threatening allergic reactions, a blood test or skin prick test is recommended.

For those looking to reduce body fat, maintain muscle mass, improve insulin sensitivity, support cardiovascular health, or promote longevity, intermittent fasting can be a helpful tool. Where most dietary interventions focus on what food is eaten, intermittent fasting is more concerned about when food is consumed. This way of eating is not new. Before agriculture, humans were hunters and gatherers who evolved to survive prolonged periods without eating. Increases in portion sizes, access to technology 24/7, and continual snacking opportunities contribute to excess caloric intake and less activity, leading to an increased risk of type 2 diabetes, heart disease, or other preventable illnesses. Intermittent fasting works by extending the period of time the body has to utilize the calories consumed from the last meal to use fat for fuel. Several intermittent fasting techniques can be used to fit personal preferences. The most popular and likely most effortless to stick to is the 16/8 fast, where one fasts for 16 hours a day and eats within eight hours. Another fasting method is the 5:2 fasting approach that involves regularly eating five days and reducing caloric intake to 500-600 calories per day on two non- consecutive days a week. A 24-hour fast one day a week is a third method that may be a little more difficult to complete. During the fasting phase, most of the time will be spent asleep, but water, tea, and coffee are permitted. Although this diet style focuses on the timing of meals, that doesn't mean it is free during the feeding phase. This method is not sustainable for those with a history of disordered eating, pregnant or breastfeeding women, or anyone under 18.

Nutrition is a continuously evolving science that can make initiating change confusing and overwhelming. Falling back on the basics of a balanced whole- foods approach with minimally processed foods continues to hold steady for positive health outcomes. Yet, the need is clear for research and guidelines around diversifying diets that are more culturally inclusive and which may therefore positively affect the health outcomes of oppressed populations. Our culture, education, medical history, unique personal preferences, socioeconomic status, and geographic location all influence our dietary choices and need to be considered when deciding what goes on one's plate.

Creating resilience through the fundamentals of health will lay a solid foundation to build one's health journey. Although the fundamentals of stress management, restorative sleep, and balanced nutrition are universally important, finding the proper technique that resonates within to achieve optimal amounts of each is a personal journey. The aim is to create autonomy and power for the individual to actively participate in their wellness. Practice and repetition will allow those techniques to become easily accessible tools in your education on how your body works and be mindful of how your body navigates the world. Listen to your body. Take notes. And, above all else, have compassion for yourself and others.

To learn more from Dr. Mullane, visit her website at lanaemullane.com

WORK CITED

American Psychological Association. (2016, March 10). Stress in America: The impact of discrimination. https://www.apa.org/news/press/releases/stress/2015/impact-of- discrimination.pdf.

Centers for Disease Control and Prevention. (2017, May 2). CDC - data and statistics - sleep and sleep disorders. Centers for Disease Control and Prevention. https://www.cdc.gov/sleep/data_statistics.html.

Chang AM, Aeschbach D, Duffy JF, Czeisler CA. (2015). Evening use of light-emitting eReaders negatively affects sleep, circadian timing, and nextmorning alertness. Proc Natl Acad Sci USA. 112(4):1232-1237. doi:10.1073/ pnas.1418490112

Dutko, P., Ver Ploeg, M., & Farrigan, T. (2012, August). Characteristics and Influential Factors of Food Deserts.

Ferracioli-Oda E, Qawasmi A, Bloch MH. (2013). Meta-analysis: melatonin for the treatment of primary sleep disorders. PLoS One. 8(5):e63773. doi:10.1371/ journal.pone.0063773

Rajilić-Stojanović M, de Vos WM. (2014). The first 1000 cultured species of the human gastrointestinal microbiota. FEMS Microbiol Rev. 38(5):996-1047. doi:10.1111/1574-6976.12075

Sánchez-Villegas A, Cabrera-Suárez B, Molero P, et al. (2019). Preventing the recurrence of depression with a Mediterranean diet supplemented with extra- virgin olive oil. The PREDI-DEP trial: study protocol. BMC Psychiatry.19(1):63. doi:10.1186/s12888-019-2036-4

https://www.ers.usda.gov/webdocs/publica-tions/45014/30940_err140.pdf.

The Nutrition Source. (2021, March 16). Healthy Eating Plate. https://www.hsph.harvard.edu/nutritionsource/healthy-eating-plate.

CHAPTER VIII

Personalized Nutrition
Ending the Hunt for the Right Diet

Nicole Visnic

The field of nutrition has reached transformative horizons, motivating and empowering individuals to effectively manage their health. The increase in chronic disease has society, at large, seeking solutions outside of mainstream healthcare. There is a growing dissatisfaction with the standard of care, and it is catalyzing a new movement in the healthcare industry. The era of 'diagnose and treat' is being replaced with an enthusiastic pursuit of health promotion and wellness.

The notion that food can be used as medicine has gained enough traction to become embraced beyond the circles of complementary and alternative medicine. The research associating nutrition and dietary habits with disease prevention is mounting daily. Even renowned medical institutions accept that chronic conditions like cardiovascular disease, dementia, and diabetes can be attenuated and even staved off through diet and lifestyle interventions.

The benefits of nutrition go beyond disease prevention. As Jeffrey Bland has famously said, "Food is information." The nutrients in food provide instructions to your cells—either moving you toward or away from homeostasis. Have you ever eaten too much, or consumed a meal that doesn't agree with you? The malaise you experience is a sign your system is out of balance. Foods and nutrients acutely affect how your body functions, and how you feel both mentally and physically. This concept is empowering yet also comes with a certain responsibility.

Once you learn that you can influence your health, you also realize your daily choices matter. This poses a quandary. In order to make good choices, you need to know what constitutes a healthy diet.

Through the decades we've seen new dietary trends surface, only to change as quickly as the seasons. Government agencies encourage us to eat a balanced diet using MyPlate. Medical doctors recommend we cut the fat, cholesterol, or carbs from our diets. Nutrition influencers promote popular diets. Each diet comes with claims to help you feel better, lose weight, and live longer. Yet there is no consensus and barely a common thread between dietary recommendations. Without unifying principles, you might feel as if you have more questions than answers. The information in this chapter is designed to provide a framework to reduce confusion, and to help you identify a way of eating that supports good health.

The Universal Diet Doesn't Exist

The idea that there is one diet that's right for everyone is a myth. Nutritional needs are as unique as the individual, and there are numerous factors that influence your needs:

- Age
- Gender
- Health conditions
- Medications
- Physical activity level
- Food intolerances
- Genetics
- Environmental stressors like industrial chemicals
- Geography
- Cultural and social factors

- Psychological stress
- Pregnancy and lactation

This list is by no means all-inclusive, but it does provide a glimpse into variables that influence your nutritional needs. At this point, it goes without saying: a universal diet cannot comprehensively address these numerous variables.

Even if you buy into the premise that there isn't one right diet for everyone, you might wonder if there is a prefab diet that is right for you. Surely, you or someone you know has benefited from a popular diet. Indeed, trialing different diets can lead you toward a way of eating that helps you feel better. It can also serve as a first step toward personalizing a diet that optimizes your health and prepares you to make adjustments, when needed. Due to the ever-evolving nature of our physiology, and the factors that influence function, our nutritional needs can change like the Nwind. Personalized nutrition allows you flexibility and freedom to make changes when your current diet no longer serves you.

What is Personalized Nutrition?

Personalized nutrition accounts for an individual's biopsychosocial construct and evaluates inter-individual differences related to the metabolism and response of nutrients. Expressed more simply, personalized nutrition is adapting diet to individual needs.

Is there any evidence that personalized diets are superior to public health diets, for instance Dietary Approaches to Stop Hypertension (DASH Diet)? You might wonder if it's worth exploring personalized nutrition when you could just follow an evidence-based diet or a diet with a successful track record. Not only is there evidence to support personalized nutrition, but the emerging research is revolutionizing the nutrition field.

A 2015 randomized control study showed personalized diets can modify postprandial elevations in blood glucose and the associated metabolic consequences The 800-person cohort was found to have high variability in the response to identical meals, suggesting that universal dietary recommendations may have limited utility. The study used a machine-learning algorithm that integrated blood parameters, dietary habits, anthropometrics (systematic measurement of the human body's physical properties), physical activity, and gut microbiota. The algorithm accurately predicts personalized postprandial glycemic responses to real-life meals (Zeevi, 2015). Consider the implications! If blood glucose can be predicted using personalized data, reductionist tools like the glycemicindex become antiquated.

Turning away from glucose control and toward lipid management, a 2010 study concluded that whole grain wheat sourdough bread influences cholesterol and triglycerides depending on genotype. In participants with the APO E3/E3 genotype, there was a significant increase in LDL cholesterol, triglycerides, and elevated ratios of HDL to triglycerides when consuming sourdough bread. Even more compelling is the fact that participants' blood sugar control was taken into consideration, an established risk factor. Genotype had even more influence on lipids than elevated blood sugar (Tucker, 2010). Clearly, both examples denote individual differences in response to the same foods. With many other studies revealing the same concept, we can now shift toward a more nuanced and meaningful nutritional paradigm. Even though personalized nutrition is in its infancy, enough information is available to make more informed decisions about how to eat for health.

Designing Your Personalized Diet in Six Steps

Step One: Building the Foundation

Every human being has basic needs for macronutrients, micronutrients, and energy/ calories. A diverse, whole-food diet is necessary to meet these needs. Whole foods should form the foundation of your diet. There is a symbiotic relationship between the nutrients contained in whole foods that work together to promote health. Take, for example, an apple. One medium apple contains about 6 mg of vitamin C; however, the other antioxidants contained in the apple, such as flavonoids and catechins, produce as much antioxidant activity as 1,500 mg of vitamin C alone.

Almonds are another great example of nutrient synergy. The flavonoids found in almond skins synergize with vitamin E found in the almond meat and more than double the antioxidant power than either of the nutrients separately (Mateljan, 2007). Nature simply cannot be replicated in the lab!

While whole-foods provide the ideal foundation for a healthy diet, there is also a place for processed foods. The primary benefit of processed foods in our harried culture is convenience and time savings. A diet composed entirely of homemade meals might seem tedious at a time when ready-to-eat food is abundantly available. Why make your own yogurt, steak sauce, or tortillas, when you can simply purchase them? A semi-homemade diet can be nutritious and support good health, but there is a caveat. You want to select products that are minimally processed. Minimally processed foods do not have refined ingredients, but rather combined ingredients; for example, take minimally processed granola. When you read the ingredient list you will see a list

183

of whole foods such as nuts, seeds, whole grains, and unrefined sweeteners like raw honey. If the ingredient list contains derivatives of whole foods or non-food ingredients, it fails the criteria for minimally processed.

A diverse diet may be just as important as consuming whole foods. The more varied your diet, the greater your chances of consuming adequate micronutrients, phytonutrients, and plant compounds with prebiotic effects. Until recently, our choices of food were dependent on seasonal availability—a natural way of diversifying and rotating the foods we eat. Evidence also suggests that a diverse diet promotes a healthy immune system, and prevents the development of food allergies (especially when started early in life) (D'Auria, 2020).

Diverse, Whole-foods Diet Checklist

1. Take a look inside your pantry and refrigerator. Is your diet made up of at least 80% whole-foods or minimally processed foods?
2. Are you rotating and diversifying your diet on a daily or weekly basis? Are you eating seasonally?

Step Two: Ancestral Diets

A diverse, whole-food diet alone can bring about significant improvements in health; however, there is another layer that deserves attention. Before modern farming and food manufacturing, human beings consumed foods native to their geographic location. The revolutionary work of a dentist named Weston Price revealed the importance not only of eating locally, but eating according to ancestry, too.

Dr. Price was perplexed by the deteriorating state of his patients' oral health and facial structures. Crowded, crooked teeth, overbites, pinched nostrils, narrowed faces, and undefined cheekbones proved common. His curiosity led him to travel to remote parts of the world about 60 years ago to investigate whether the problems he was observing in his patients were a collective problem. What he found were tribes and villages where virtually every individual exhibited robust health. Tooth decay was rare, dental crowding and occlusions non-existent. The natives were invariably good natured and characterized by impressive physical development with virtually no signs of disease. He photographed the tribes and recorded his observations in the landmark book, Nutrition & Physical Degeneration (Price, 2003).

A particularly interesting finding in Price's research was the disparity in diets of indigenous populations. In fact, their diets varied as much as popular trends today. In the Swiss village where Price began his diverse investigations, the inhabitants lived on rich dairy products, rye bread, occasional meat, bone broth soups, and the few vegetables they could cultivate during summer months. In Alaska, the Eskimo diet was composed largely of fish and marine animals, including seal oil and blubber. Tribes in Canada, the Everglades, the Amazon, Australia and Africa consumed game animals, organ meats, glands, blood, marrow, a variety of grains, tubers, and seasonal vegetables and fruits. Price's findings provide revelatory clues about the significance of ancestry and eating foods native to one's geographical location as it relates to good health and prevention of disease. The only problem is most of us are transplanted from our origin of ancestry and do not come from a homogeneous gene pool. This immediately raises the question, how could you possibly apply this information?

To refine your diet based on ancestral principles, you want to prioritize consumption of locally grown food, and minimize foods that were not a part of any ancestral diet. Foods that have been grown and raised locally are more nutritious, whereas imported foods lose nutrients rapidly during transportation. There are many studies demonstrating the micronutrient depletion that occurs postharvest. One study found a significant decrease in ascorbic acid, total chlorophyll content, and carotenoids found in lettuce heads within days of harvest. The ascorbic acid lost from lettuce by the time it arrived on the retail shelf was 48% by day three, and 68.9% by day four (Managa, 2018). One of the attractions of eating nutritious foods is to obtain micronutrients and phytonutrients. If the food you're buying has lost vital nutrients during transportation, you're missing out on the very compounds you're intending to consume. There are several ways to begin introducing local foods into your diet:

- Local farmer's market
- CSA (Community-supported agriculture), subscribing to/paying for a share of local harvests
- Purchasing local produce at your supermarket
- Growing some of your own food. Herb gardens and microgreen quilts are a great place to start!

In addition to eating locally, you can also move closer to an ancestral diet by limiting consumption of food products that didn't exist before industrial food manufacturing. Adulterated foods tend to lack nutrients and the synergistic complexity of whole foods. They also possess properties that can interfere with normal function. Refined sugar, solvent-extracted cooking oils, fractionated grains, and artificial ingredients were never a part of our early ancestor diets. Those same ingredients are also absent in the diets of populations living in Blue Zones, our best epidemiological evidence for achieving health and longevity.

Ancestral Diet Checklist

1. On a weekly basis are you visiting your local farmer's market, ordering from a CSA, or gathering food from your garden?
2. Does your diet resemble the diet of your great grandparents?

Step Three: Biopsychosocial Influence

At this point it might seem as if healthy eating can be accomplished through moderation, and choosing seasonal, locally grown foods. Healthy eating, however, is much more than eating the right foods, at the right time of year, and from the right location. If healthy eating was as simple as following the guidelines in steps one and two, everyone would be doing it! Personalized nutrition extends beyond food and accounts for psychosocial elements. It addresses variables that influence your dietary choices and the way these variables alter your responses to food.

There is a dynamic confluence among your diet, inner world, and social sphere that deserves just as much attention as the foods you eat. Let's first start with some of the factors that affect your dietary choices. Throughout the day, we experience shifts in our mental-emotional state, and encounter circumstances that affect us in varying degrees. We are not always cognizant of the contributing factors.

- Eating (or not eating) for emotional reasons
- Low energy and motivation to prioritize healthy eating
- Reliance on take-out or processed foods due to time limitations
- Lack of culinary skills or lack of interest in learning how to cook
- Dietary habits of those within your household or peer group

- Changes to your routine, such as travel
- Exceptions to your routine, such as special occasions
- Business or social meals
- The influence of news and social media

Without presumption of these psychosocial influences, you would be missing the forest through the trees. Simply becoming aware of this concept allows you to think more expansively about dietary adherence. The primary reason most people fail to adopt healthy eating patterns is because they rely on willpower, not realizing compliance is much more than self-discipline. As a biopsychosocial being, you are more like the ecology of an ocean than the mechanics of a computer. When you realize how complex and non-linear behavior change is, you are able to adjust your expectations and set more realistic goals.

Psychosocial influence is not limited to dietary adherence; it also impacts our biology. One of the ways this occurs is through the gut-brain axis (GBA): "The GBA consists of bidirectional communication between your central nervous system and your enteric nervous system, linking emotional and cognitive centers of the brain with peripheral intestinal functions" (Carabotti, 2015). This means your psychology affects your gut and your gut affects your psychology.

Have you ever felt nervous and experienced butterflies in your stomach? This is a brain-gut interaction that occurs as a result of a stress response. Blood vessels to the gut constrict and digestive muscles contract leading to a fluttering sensation. Now consider eating a meal when you are experiencing restricted blood flow and muscle contractions. Ultimately, your gastrointestinal system is forced to function within a physiological state that's unfavorable for digestion. This can lead to obvious symptoms of indigestion or asymptomatic shifts in your microbiome and gut function.

The parasympathetic nervous system is the side of your nervous system that facilitates normal digestion. It is responsible for rest-and-digest functions. The more relaxed and content you are, the better your digestion and overall health. Life stressors are a normal part of living, but there are ways to feel more at ease and to prime your digestion for meal time.

- Take a moment before eating to think of someone or something you appreciate.
- Slow your respiration rate by taking a few diaphragmatic breaths.
- Eat slowly and chew your food until it is the consistency of baby food.
- When possible, dine with people who lift your spirits.

Biopsychosocial Checklist

1. Are you aware of the psychosocial factors that influence your dietary choices? If so, are you addressing or accounting for those variables?
2. Do you regularly practice good meal hygiene to optimize digestion and gut function?

Step Four: Biochemical Individuality

Now that you have foundational principles for creating a personalized diet, it's appropriate to segue into a more nuanced approach to nutrition. Biochemical individuality is the concept that the nutritional and biochemical constitution of each person is unique and that dietary needs vary from person to person.

In 1956, the late world-renowned biochemist Roger Williams, Ph.D., published his book **Biochemical Individuality (Williams, 1975)**, in which he describes anatomical and physiological differences among people and how the variations relate to individual responses to the environment. Williams was one of the first to recognize how biochemical individuality related to differing nutritional needs for good health. Williams gives an example in his book illustrating the genetic impact associated with potassium, a mineral tightly regulated in the blood. The most convincing evidence that there is substantial variation in the potassium needs of human individuals is the existence of familial periodic paralysis which is accompanied by low potassium levels. In afflicted individuals, the potassium level prior to seizure is 2.6 to 3.0 meq per liter and relief of the condition comes promptly after administration of 2 to 5 grams of potassium chloride. The disease is thought to be due to inherited needs for higher amounts of potassium, possibly due to differences in enzyme systems and excretion rates.

Differing nutrient levels, and nutrient needs, are not unique to potassium. The same evidence exists for nearly every micronutrient, macronutrient, amino acid, and fatty acid. Since nutrient needs vary from person to person, the diet that promotes good health in one individual will be different from the diet that promotes good health in another. You may have experienced this phenomenon yourself. Perhaps a friend of yours changed their diet and experienced symptom reduction or weight loss, but when trying the same diet, you didn't have the same response. This is completely normal, and now, you can understand why. Initially, this concept may cause more confusion. You're probably wondering how you could possibly figure out how to eat based on your unique biochemical individuality.

This topic is vast and it could take an entire lifetime to unravel the complex interplay between diet and inter-individual differences; however, there is a road map to help guide you. By gathering biometrics and using biofeedback, you can begin customizing your diet based on your unique needs.

Biochemical Individuality: Clinical Labs

Your physician or healthcare provider can and should run comprehensive clinical labs every year. Clinical lab data allow you to evaluate the effects of your current diet and lifestyle, identify genetic predispositions, and gain information to guide personalized nutrition recommendations.

Your comprehensive labs should include:

- Complete Blood Count (CBC)
- Comprehensive Metabolic Panel (CMP)
- Advanced lipid testing
- Glucose metabolism markers
- Sex hormones
- Thyroid hormones and thyroid antibodies
- Adrenal hormones
- Uric acid
- Homocysteine
- Prolactin
- Vitamin D
- Iron and ferritin
- hsCRP

Each of these markers provides clues about your health, and each has nutritional implications. Nutritional interventions can either have a direct impact on biomarkers or play a supportive role in balancing your biochemistry. Let's take a look at a few examples.

Homocysteine is an independent risk factor for cardiovascular disease. When homocysteine is elevated, it indicates impaired methylation and/or recycling. There are several reasons for these impairments, but simply taking nutrients like L-5- methyltetrahydrofolate (folate), methylcobalamin (vitamin B12), and pyridoxal-5- phosphate (vitamin B6), allows homocysteine to be properly converted or recycled. These nutrients directly lower homocysteine and help reduce your risk for heart disease.

Uric acid is another example of a biomarker that can be directly affected by diet. Uric acid is a metabolic waste product of purines (the building blocks of RNA and DNA). Elevated uric acid is most commonly associated with gout, but is also a risk factor for metabolic syndrome. Uric acid can be lowered by consuming adequate water and reducing alcohol, purine-rich foods, and fructose. In addition to lowering uric acid, there are nutritional factors that improve uric acid metabolism, such as vitamin C, cherries, and dietary fiber. Whether uric acid is elevated for dietary reasons or inflammatory reasons (e.g. infection or injury), nutritional interventions play a role in normalizing levels.

Now, let's examine the way nutrition plays a supportive role in adrenal health. Cortisol is an adrenal hormone with many functions. One of its primary roles is to activate the stress response. When you experience stress, whether real or perceived, your adrenal glands release cortisol to prepare you for fight or flight–a well-orchestrated physiological cascade. Unfortunately, chronic stress disrupts normal adrenal function leading to many symptoms, one of those being loss of glycemic control. This is because one of cortisol's roles is to raise blood sugar. When cortisol is constantly elevated, there are changes that reduce hormone availability and efficacy, and dips in blood sugar start to occur. By supporting your blood sugar with regularly spaced meals, you can reduce some of the demand on your adrenal glands.

Infrequent meals and fasting are analogous to whipping a tired horse. Cortisol will eventually get the job done, but it comes with a cost and exacerbates the existing dysfunction.

Clinical labs provide a tremendous amount of information that can guide personalized nutrition recommendations. Given the technical nature of clinical labs, it would be wise to work with a healthcare provider who has experience in clinical nutrition. There are also plenty of educational resources available that help decode the relationship between nutrition and biomarkers.

Biochemical Individuality: Genetic Testing

Genomic profiling is now a reality, and many individuals have already taken advantage of the technology. Genomic profiling is a comprehensive and informative analysis of tens of thousands of genes providing information on ancestry, medication tolerance, disease risk, and much more—including how to eat. Over the years there have been several genediet interactions established.

- Lactose Tolerance. Decreased activity of the LCT gene inhibits production of lactase, an enzyme that breaks down lactose. Individuals with decreased LCT activity who consume lactose containing foods like milk, yogurt, cheese, and ice cream typically experience digestive symptoms like gas, bloating, abdominal cramping, and diarrhea.

193

- Caffeine Metabolism. Possessing even one copy of the CYP1A2*1F gene reduces caffeine metabolism. Slow caffeine metabolizers who consume caffeine are at greater risk for heart conditions and myocardial infarction. Caffeine consumption in slow metabolizers is also associated with infertility and miscarriages.

- Lipid Metabolism. The APOE gene affects how you metabolize and transport fats and cholesterol throughout your body. Individuals with a certain variation of the APOE gene, known as APOE4, tend to have higher levels of LDL and increased risk for metabolic syndrome and Alzheimer's when consuming a diet high in saturated fat and refined carbohydrates.

- Micronutrient Utilization. One of the most well-known genediet interactions is with the MTHFR gene. Individuals with a variation in this gene are unable to efficiently utilize folic acid and require supplementation with a methylated form of folate. Without proper supplementation, individuals with this variation are at increased risk for heart disease, cancer, mood disorders, and having children with neural tube defects.

As you can see, your genes influence the way you metabolize and respond to nutrients and dietary compounds. Epigenetics is a process by which external factors change the expression of your genes. This is one of the reasons a personalized diet and lifestyle approach is essential.

The choices you make influence the expression of your genes, either offering protection or increasing risk for disease. This is empowering information when applied correctly. When considering genetic profiling, it's important to select a test that provides actionable recommendations. Genetic testing is only as useful as your ability to decrease risk. Testing genes with limited gene-nutrient research has little relevance and no utility. This is an area of nutrition that can create more confusion than clarity. Working with a professional who has expertise interpreting and applying nutrigenomics within the context of your overall health is worth the investment.

Biochemical Individuality: Microbiome

At the heart of biochemical individuality is the microbiome, an entire ecosystem of microorganisms residing on and within our bodies. Your microbiome is as unique as your fingerprint, but infinitely more complex. You have trillions of microorganisms harmoniously coexisting and communicating with the cells and genes of your body, orchestrating essential biological functions.

Gut microbes influence gastrointestinal, immune, and metabolic health. They also influence neurobehavioral traits (Valdes, 2018). The most abundant microbes are present in the colon. Commensal bacteria (indigenous bacteria) have many health- promoting functions. Some of those functions include the following:

- Provide a physical barrier in the GI tract to protect the epithelium
- Prevent foreign invaders from entering circulation
- Produce substances to destroy viruses, fungus, and pathogenic bacteria
- Neutralize metabolic byproducts and toxic substances
- Inactivate histamine, chelate heavy metals, and absorb carcinogens
- Synthesize B vitamins and vitamin K
- Produce short chain fatty acids

Once you realize the magnitude by which commensal bacteria influence health, it becomes possible to understand the relationship between microbiome and disease. Deranged gut bacteria are associated with many multifactorial diseases, including IBD, autoimmune diseases, eczema, autism, psychiatric disorders, periodontal disease, atherosclerosis, allergies, colon cancer, and obesity.

Robust health hinges on a balanced and diverse microbial terrain. This is where eating a diverse, whole-foods diet shines. Whole foods contain compounds like prebiotics, polyphenols, probiotics, and omega 3 fatty acids. These compounds have been shown to influence microbial diversity.

- Prebiotics are found in foods like garlic, onion, leeks, asparagus, chicory, Jerusalem artichoke, green bananas, and edamame.
- Polyphenols are found in foods like green tea, cinnamon, cloves, citrus, berries, pomegranate, grapes, flaxseeds, and oats.
- Probiotics are found in fermented and cultured foods like sauerkraut, kimchi, yogurt, kefir, miso, and natto.
- Omega 3 fatty acids are found in foods like salmon, trout, herring, anchovies, sardines, flaxseeds, algae, and chia seeds.

If you are unaccustomed to eating prebiotic and probiotics foods, it's important you incorporate these foods into your diet gradually to prevent gastrointestinal stress. Prebiotic foods in particular have potent effects and your microbiome needs time to acclimate to their effects. Ironically, prebiotic and probiotic foods can worsen symptoms in individuals who have digestive conditions like IBS and small intestine bacterial overgrowth (SIBO). These conditions have a common thread of dysbiosis and require special diets until the underlying cause is addressed.

Personalized nutrition cannot be overstated when addressing dysbiotic conditions. Two individuals with the same condition, SIBO for instance, tend to respond differently to a low fermentation diet (a condition- specific diet). This is because condition-specific models error on the side of generalization, i.e. what works for a group will work for the individual.

As a clinical nutritionist, I spend most of my time working with clients who have functional gastrointestinal disorders. The limitations of condition-specific models are obvious when dealing with refractory conditions. Complex health conditions tend to be recalcitrant for all the reasons listed in the biochemical individuality section. A case-based paradigm, in contrast, broadens the tool kit. Solving complicated problems requires critical thinking, finesse, innovation, and above all, attention to biochemical individuality.

Biochemical Individuality Checklist

3. Do you have an annual check-up with a healthcare provider to evaluate clinical labs? If so, are you making changes to improve values outside the reference range?
4. Are you incorporating foods with prebiotics, probiotics, polyphenol, and omega 3 fatty acids to help nourish your microbiome?
5. Bonus: Have you done genetic testing to identify gene-nutrient risk factors like MTHFR?

Step Five: Family History

With a basic understanding of gene-nutrient interactions and biopsychosocial influence, it becomes possible to put family history into proper context. Family history is arguably the most important tool for stratifying disease risk. The majority of chronic conditions are the result of a complex interplay between numerous genetic variants and environmental factors. Family history is a significant predictor of future disease because of the overlapping factors between you and your family, such as genetic variants, shared environment, familial dietary habits, and common behaviors.

It is worth noting that family history should not be considered outside the context of epigenetics? Reducing disease-risk to family history alone becomes deterministic rather than modifiable. The development of disease is a multifactorial process with many interventional avenues for prevention. If early heart disease runs in your family, you could be tempted to believe it's an inheritable disease. Research, on the other hand, shows that heart disease is the result of numerous factors that extend beyond genetic predisposition. Taking an ecological viewpoint versus a deterministic viewpoint would allow you to see familial patterns that increase or decrease risk for heart disease.

- Does your family eat enough fiber, polyphenolic compounds, omega 3 fatty acids, magnesium-rich foods?
- Are their vitamin K2 levels optimal?
- How often does your family eat homemade meals?
- Do their waist-to-hip measurements fall within the healthy range?
- Is alcohol consumption within the CDC's guidelines?
- Do they have other conditions associated with inflammation?
- How well does your family manage stress?
- What is your family's physical activity level? Do they meet the exercise requirements for heart health?

The first step in reducing disease risk is to do an inventory of the diseases prevalent in your family: great grandparents, grandparents, parents, aunts, uncles, and siblings. Once you have this information you can begin to assess your risk using clinical lab tests and biometric tests like blood pressure and waist-to-hip circumference.

The second step is analyzing your clinical labs and biometric tests. Say for instance you have elevated LDL-P, triglycerides, and homocysteine. Each of these markers increases risk for heart disease and each can be modified to a certain degree using nutritional interventions.

Once assessing clinical labs and biometric tests, you can go a step further and use genetic tests to gain more information and direction. If you have one or two APOE E4 alleles, your risk for heart disease increases. Because the E4 allele is associated with impaired lipid metabolism, you can leverage the information to minimize dietary risk factors associated with deranged lipids.

Retest your values after 12 weeks of diet modification to determine how much the intervention modified your biomarkers. Your results will either confirm you're on the right track or let you know the plan needs to be adjusted.

Family History Checklist

- Have you done an inventory of your family's health history?
- Are you aware of diet, lifestyle, or behavioral patterns associated with increased risk for disease?

Step Six: Biofeedback

One of the most valuable tools in personalized nutrition is biofeedback. Biofeedback is the way your body communicates with you to promote self-preservation. Utilizing biofeedback allows you to leverage your body's innate wisdom and modify your behavior to protect your health. There are objective and subjective forms of biofeedback. Vital signs and biometrics are forms of objective biofeedback. Elevated heart rate and respiration rate, for instance, indicate sympathetic arousal. Symptoms, or changes in well-being, are subjective forms of biofeedback. If you experience indigestion every time you eat jalapeno peppers, the symptom indicates a food incompatibility. Your body doesn't just alert you to potential danger, it also reveals what it needs. If you spend time with friends and your craving for ice cream vanishes, it's an indicator you need more connection time. If you start meditating and experience an improvement in sleep, it's an indicator you need more relaxation or restoration.

Using biofeedback may seem like common sense, yet people do not embrace it for a number of reasons. Those with busy and demanding lives tend to disassociate from symptoms. Noticing symptoms and correlations interferes with productivity. It seems more efficient to ignore symptoms and press on. There is also a category of people who don't trust their body's feedback or would rather defer to someone they think knows better. External validation seems more reliable than their intuition. Another reason people dismiss biofeedback is because there is a payoff to certain behaviors. Giving up favorite foods or alcohol, for instance, doesn't seem worth the sacrifice.

Health is built on pattern detection. Paying attention to variables that impact your health or well-being makes it possible to intervene. Generally, the sooner you take action, the greater your odds of preventing unnecessary health challenges. The same goes for factors that enhance well-being. Consistently attending to your biopsychosocial needs improves your healthspan. Biofeedback is highly useful when assessing whether you're on the right track with your diet. When you're eating in a way that balances your body chemistry, you should feel stable after meals. If you experience fatigue, cravings, indigestion, appetite issues, or any other symptom, it's a sign you need to make adjustments. One way to identify the right fuel for your engine is by experimenting with two contrasting meals.

Let's say you eat Greek yogurt and granola for breakfast, and an hour after the meal you experience sugar cravings and hunger. The next morning, try a meal with a totally different macronutrient composition, like eggs and smoked salmon. If you are free of cravings and your hunger is under control until lunch, you've identified the right fuel. The meal that maintains homeostasis is generally the meal that supports your health.

Your body's feedback should be the supreme authority when evaluating

whether your diet is working for you. It can be difficult to accept this at a time when there is excessive external pressure to eat a certain way. We are inundated with headlines that influence our perspective on healthy eating. If the research shows broccoli helps prevent cancer, but you feel bloated and gaseous after eating it, it's in your best interest to stop eating it. Only you know whether dietary changes are making you feel better or worse. Research and experts can provide insight and guidance, but it's ultimately up to you to determine whether you're on the right path.

Personalized nutrition is a framework that allows you to adjust your diet according to your individual needs and responses to food. Cultivating a diet that's right for you can be basic, e.g. using biofeedback to make adjustments to a diverse, whole-foods diet. It can also be multilayered, e.g. utilizing genetic profiling and comprehensive clinical labs to refine your diet. In some ways personalized nutrition is like a game of chess. By making strategic moves, you gain leverage over risk factors and favorably influence the trajectory of your health and your quality of life.

WORKS CITED

Carabotti, M., Scirocco, A., Maselli, M. A., & Severi, C. (2015). The gut-brain axis: interactions between enteric microbiota, central and enteric nervous systems. Annals of gastroenterology, 28(2), 203–209.

D'Auria, E., Peroni, D. G., Sartorio, M., Verduci, E., Zuccotti, G. V., & Venter, NC. (2020). The Role of Diet Diversity and Diet Indices on Allergy Outcomes.

Frontiers in pediatrics, 8, 545. https://doi.org/10.3389/fped.2020.00545
Kosower, N., Rein, M., Zilberman-Schapira, G., Dohnalová, L., Pevsner-Fischer, M., Bikovsky,R., … Segal, E. (2015). Personalized Nutrition by Prediction of Glycemic Responses. Cell, 163(5), 1079 1094. https://doi.org/10.1016/j.cell.2015.11.001

Lador, D., Avnit-Sagi, T., Lotan-Pompan, M., Suez, J., Mahdi, J. A., Matot, E., Malka, G.,Tucker AJ, Mackay KA, Robinson LE, Graham TE, Bakovic M,Duncan AM. "The effect of whole grain wheat sourdough bread consumptionon serum lipids in healthy normoglycemic/normoinsulinemic and hyperglycemic/hyperinsulinemic adults depends on presence of the APOE E3/E3 genotype:a randomized controlled trial." Nutr Metab (Lond). 2010 May 5; 7:37.doi: 10.1186/1743-7075-7-37. PMID: 20444273; PMCID: PMC2877680.

Managa, M. G., Tinyani, P. P., Senyolo, G. M., Soundy, P., Sultanbawa, Y., &Sivakumar, D. (2018). Impact of transportation, storage, and retail shelf conditionson lettuce quality and phytonutrients losses in the supply chain. Food science & nutrition, 6(6), 1527–1536. https://doi.org/10.1002/fsn3.685

Mateljan, George (2007). World's Healthiest Foods. The George Mateljan Foundation. Price, W. A., & Price-Pottenger Nutrition Foundation. (2003). Nutrition and physical degeneration. La Mesa, CA: Price-Pottenger Nutrition Foundation

Williams, R. J. (1975). Biochemical individuality. University of Texas Press.

Valdes, A. M., Walter, J., Segal, E., & Spector, T. D. (2018). Role of the gutmicrobiota in nutrition and health. BMJ (Clinical research ed.), 361, k2179.
https://doi.org/10.1136/bmj.k2179.
Zeevi, D., Korem, T., Zmora, N., Israeli, D., Rothschild, D., Weinberger, A., Ben-Yacov, O.,

"Personalized Nutrition by Prediction of Glycemic Responses." Cell, V. 163, Issue 5, November 2015, 1079-1094. 173

CHAPTER IX

Universal Touch: Untangling Patterns, Awakening Awareness

Maria Santoro

"And the day came when the risk it took to remain tight in a bud was more painful than the risk it took to blossom."
-Anaïs Nin

Most of what we think about life comes from a set of assumptions we have been taught, which we often don't examine or even question. Medical paradigms are what determine how we think about our bodies. Over the years, our medical paradigm in the West has been shifting and advancing. We have learned more about mind-body connections giving rise to new methods of treatment and healing.

The emphasis of this book is the interconnectedness of all systems and modalities used to treat and heal the body. While my focus is massage therapy, no one system, treatment or modality can fully address each pain, restriction, weakness or strength in the body.

My main goal of this chapter is to help the reader understand not only how the living body works, but how human biology can be linked to broader considerations of how a human exists within, interacts with their environment, and experiences existence in emotional, spiritual as well as physical terms and to understand the applications, benefits and mechanisms of bodywork.

As a licensed massage therapist, trained in both Eastern and Western traditions, I use all modalities from Swedish, medical massage, deep tissue, manual lymphatic drainage (MLD), ART(Active Release Technique), myofascial release, myofascial unwinding, craniosacral, Shiatsu, Watsu, Thai massage, Mayan abdominal massage to reflexology in my practice. While all of these modalities are invaluable, each one has its unique function in treatment. I will in this chapter focus on those which through my experience and training I feel most connect the mind and body using a whole system approach, I am not promoting one technique over another nor even positing a mechanism for how any one technique works. What is of utmost importance is understanding that the heart of all treatment lies in our ability to listen, to perceive, to see more than in our application of technique. Comprehend the bigger picture of your own or your client's structural relationships, then apply whatever technique you have learned toward resolving that pattern. We are all different, yet we are all alike. Everyone on this earth is a work in progress, from the finely tuned athlete to the physically challenged. We all possess the ability to exceed our limits once we recognize what they are and learn to embrace the process as much as the result. To have been given the privilege of assisting one in their process has been for me the most rewarding gift.

THE TIES THAT BIND

The human body is the most enchanting and fascinating of all creations. It is an intricate web of fascia wrapping around millions and millions of cells making up all the systems of the body, each functioning in its own unique way to keep us in this complex dance we call homeostasis. The skin, the skeleton, joints and muscles, the heart and circulatory system, the lymphatic system, the lungs, the gut, the kidneys and bladder, the nervous system, the special senses and the reproductive system cannot and do not function alone. Even though each cell has its individual life function, there is always coherence. We are an integrated whole, not a sum of our parts.

In the West, the prevailing traditional paradigm that you and I were taught is the Cartesian/Newtonian model of reality, and it is over three hundred years old. This model of classic physics which is the basis of our current paradigm "proposes to analyze the phenomena from the analogy of a machine," where knowing the operation of the isolated parts is able to understand the whole formed by those parts.

Newton and Descartes both believed there was a fundamental divide between mind and matter; that is, between mental and physical processes. In the field of medical science, this paradigm has reduced human illness to the "biochemistry of disease," completely losing sight of the fact that disease or dysfunction is part of a whole system including the

mind and the natural environment we live in. Essentially, what they are saying is that brain function, and emotions of fear, sorrow, anger, joy are nothing more than chemical reactions (Kurtz, R.). This separatist mechanistic approach to life, which is brilliant in its own way, lacks a connection between the mind, body and spirit, between a person and their environment, overlooking the fact that there is an intelligence running through the body connecting all.

The mainstream mechanistic view is that the brain is responsible for what we in the West call the "mind." As useful as it has been, it has objectified rather than humanized our relationship to our insides. As we incorporate more quantum physics into biology, more has been discovered about what makes us tick. The mind is understood to be not only in the brain, but everywhere in a network of flow of communication in the tissues of the body as well as the brain.

ROOTS

My introduction to massage techniques and understanding of the body as an integrated whole began in an Eastern tradition while I was living abroad in Asia. It was in Korea that I was first introduced to a book called the "Dongui Bogam," a Korean book compiled by the royal physician Heo Jun and first published in 1613 during the Joseon Dynasty of Korea. The book has been listed as one of the national treasures of South Korea and is registered with UNESCO. The title literally means **"a priceless book about medicine of an Eastern country."** Its innovative disease classification system is based on essence, Qi (energy), and spirit, and its emphasis is on the importance of disease prevention through the promotion of health regimens. Introducing a unique and pragmatic form of medicine, the Dongui Bogam regards the human body as a universe and understands body function, health maintenance, and the treatment of disease according to comprehensive and systematic approaches. It also states that humans are emotional creatures. We communicate and make relationships by expressing our feelings; when not properly released, these emotions are linked to illness and restrictions in the body. The book begins with the following elusive paragraph that fascinated me:

> Mankind is the most precious of all living things in the Universe. The round head resembles heaven, and the flat foot resembles earth; man has four limbs as the universe has four seasons, man has five viscera as the universe has five phases; man has six bowels as the universe has six extremes, man has eight joints as the universe has eight winds, man has nine orifices as

the universe has nine stars, and man has twelve meridians as the universe has twelve hours. Man has twenty-four acupoints as the universe has twenty-four qi. Also, man has 365 joints as the universe has 365 divisions; man has two eyes as the universe has the sun and the moon, man sleeps and wakes as the universe has day and night; man has happiness and anger as the universe has thunder and lightning, and man has tears and nasal discharge as the universe has rain and dew; man has cold and heat as the universe has yin and willpower, and man has blood vessels as the universe has spring water; man has hair growing as the universe has grass and trees; and man has teeth as the universe has metal and rocks.

This fascinating logic emphasizes that both nature and humans are created and function together —a much different view from that of the Cartesian/Newtonian model I was taught in the West. We all have our own beliefs and theory on the mental and the physical or mind and body, and mind and brain. I understand these beliefs are not without controversy or skepticism. Through my own training, teachings, and experience I have found not only that is there is a powerful connection between the mind and body, but also that we are an infinite part of our environment. We depend on it as much as we influence it. To stay healthy, one must maintain harmony within the body and adapt to the changes going on outside of it.

Teachings in the Yellow Emperor's Classic of Medicine give a holistic picture of human life. It does not separate external changes—geographic, climatic, or seasonal, for instance—from internal changes such as emotions and our responses to them. It tells how our way of life and environment affect our health. For example, "When damp invades the body, the head will feel heavy and distended, as if highly bandaged.

The large muscles and tendons will contract, and the small muscles and tendons will become flaccid, resulting in a loss of mobility, spasms, and atrophy" (Ni, 9).

It wasn't until 1977 in the West that George Engel was the first to suggest that to understand a person's medical condition it is not simply the biological factors to consider, but also the psychological and social factors. This is known as the Biopsychosocial Model and is most commonly used in chronic pain, with the view that pain is a psychophysiological pattern that cannot be categorized into biological, psychological, or social factors alone (Engel, G.).

CHRONICLE OF MASSAGE

Let's begin to understand what we have come to know today as massage with its history. Most ancient cultures practiced some form of healing touch. Healing with the hands is considered to be the oldest form of medicine. The word massage itself comes from the Arabic verb "masah," meaning to "to rub." Massage has a long history dating back to 3000 BC (or earlier) where it originated in India and was considered a sacred system of healing. It was used not only to heal injuries, relieve pain, and promote relaxation, but also to cure and treat illnesses. The Hindus in Ayurveda believe that disease is caused when people are out of sync with their environment. Massage is believed to restore the body's natural and physical balance so that it can heal naturally.

As cultures and history evolved, the healing methods of massage traveled all over the world, with all cultures putting their own spin on it. It then went on to become known by two names: Tui-Na (pushpull), and Anmo-Anma (press-rub). These methods of Chinese and Japanese origins were performed by kneading or rubbing down the entire body with the hands while using gentle pressure and traction. In the West,

Hippocrates of Cos (460-377BC) was the first physician to describe specifically the medical benefits of anointing (using oil) and massage. He called his art "anatripsis," which means to rub up. He held the belief that the body must be treated as a whole and not just as a series of parts. Massage then came to the Romans from the Greeks. Julius Cesar (100-44BC) used massage daily to relieve his neuralgia and prevent epileptic seizures. The Romans believed a healthy mind is a healthy body.

The popularity of massage declined in the West until the 17th century, when discoveries in pharmacology and medical technology advanced. Per Henrik Ling (1676-1839), a Swedish doctor who brought it out of retirement, is credited with Swedish massage, although he did not invent it. The form of massage in the West today we are most familiar with, it involves stroking, pressing, squeezing, and striking. While Ling's methods are still used today, Jonah George Mezger, a Dutchman, refined Dr. Ling's techniques and is credited with other popular techniques of massage such as effleurage, petrissage, tapotement, and friction—all techniques we still use today.

By the late 1800's, the full-body massage became part of the "rest cure" for the type of melancholy known as neurasthenia that was popular among society ladies who lived the wealthy life of the late 1800's. Even Sigmund Freud (1856-1939) experimented with massage in the treatment of hysteria, a form of mental illness that is characterized by hysteria, but has no physiological basis. In 1916, Dr James Mennell went on to use certain forms of tactile stimulation, such as stroking and light touch, mostly developed by him.

Massage is its own healing practice, and is the origin of many medical practices that later arose, such as physical therapy and chiropractic manipulation. It uses the most natural form of medicine (human touch) and transcends the particulars of human culture and history.

While our scientific knowledge has changed over the centuries, massage as an applied healing practice has not changed dramatically, just as the human body has not changed significantly. We are still using most of the modalities learned through history; as our medical paradigms shifted in the West, however, we continued to learn about and to use more whole-system approaches with massage.

THE POWER OF TOUCH

I believe we all can attest to the importance of touch. Skin to skin contact has been encouraged as soon as babies emerge from the womb. Every mother touches, holds, kisses or caresses her child when they are in pain or in need of comfort. What is the first thing we do when we hurt ourselves? Usually we touch the hurt part of our body. This physical instinct sends signals to the part that was hurt to promote healing. Skin is the largest organ in the body and is often referred to as one big sense organ. It has many sensory receptors that enable us to feel light touch, pressure, temperature, vibration, and pain. Skin contact is used to stimulate some of these receptors, leading to a particular reaction depending on which receptors are stimulated and what effect is achieved and determined by the nature of the skin contact.

Like our other senses, touch comes in gradations. An exquisite array of receptors can distinguish minute variations in the environment. Using fast, slow, deep, light, hot, cold will have different biological effects in the body. Pacinian corpuscles, one of the pressure receptors, send signals directly to a nerve bundle deep in the brain called the vagus nerve. The vagus is sometimes called "the wanderer" because it has branches that wander throughout the body to several internal organs, including the heart. It is the vagus nerve that slows heart rate down and decreases blood pressure. Some receptors react only to caress, while others send pain signals.

Each type activates a different part of the brain, making us feel soothed or hurt, comforted or distressed, angry or calm. David Linden, a Johns Hopkins neuroscientist, cites "the electric touch of romantic love, the unsettling feeling of being watched, the relief of pain from mindful practice, or the essential touch that newborns need to thrive" as diverse sensations that "flow from the evolved nature of our skin, nerves and brain" (Linden, D.).

In the mid-1970's, Tiffany Field (head of the Touch Research Institute at the University of Miami Miller School of Medicine), was a new mother. She massaged her infant daughter, who was born prematurely. The calming effects she witnessed inspired her to study prematurity and massage. The research showed that massage caused premature infants to gain more weight than their non-massaged premature infants (Field et al.). Even short bursts of touch—as little as 15 minutes in the evening— in one of her studies not only enhanced growth and weight gain in children, but also led to emotional, physical, and cognitive improvements in adults. Touch in general appears to stimulate our bodies in very specific ways (Field,T.).

Studies in Romania in the 1990s examined the sensory deprivation of children. The touch-deprived children, they found, had significantly higher cortisol levels (a stress hormone) and slower growth developments for their age group (Carlson, M.). Another study indicated that when pre-school aged kids and adolescents are touched less, they become more physically aggressive towards each other (Field,T.). Continuing to study touch, Dr. Field now is looking at the elderly.

One group of elderly participants received regular conversation-filled visits while another received social visits that also included massage; the second group saw emotional and cognitive benefits over and above those of the first. It is easy to see how an elderly person who is regularly visited by a massage therapist or who is engaging with touch in some way might be happier and healthier than one who is not. In studies with elderly people that had the elderly massage babies, versus receiving massage, interestingly enough they found the effects were greater when they were giving the massage rather than receiving. This goes to show touch is as beneficial both giving and receiving. Massage therapists are also getting some kind of benefit from stimulating the pressure receptors in the hands, elbow, or whatever body part they're massaging with.

One of the greatest losses during COVID and quarantine where people had to physically be distanced from one another definitely resulted in touch deprivation. As a massage therapist, I certainly felt it myself. In fact, a survey put together found that touch deprivation was highly correlated to anxiety symptoms to depression symptoms, to boredom and to loneliness. Every negative scale and rating on the survey was related to touch deprivation. What they also saw is that the immune system is being more compromised (Field, T.). So, as you can see, both touch and its lack affect our bodies in very specific ways.

MORE THAN JUST SKIN DEEP

I have always been enraptured by the physiological, biochemical, and emotional reactions massage promotes. The many benefits of massage include pain relief, relaxation, improved sleep quality, decreased stress and inflammation, decreased blood pressure as well as improved mental health and release of stored emotional and physical trauma. So how does all this work in the body? Let's go a little deeper and discuss some of the mechanisms and benefits of massage.

Physiological, Biochemical, and Emotional Mechanisms of Massage

- Massage using light pressure releases oxytocin, a neurotransmitter that is produced in the hypothalamus. It is known as the "love hormone" or "feel good" hormone because its levels increase during hugging and orgasm as well as massage. It also regulates our emotional responses including trust, empathy, and positive memories. Oxytocin stimulates other "feel good" hormones such as serotonin and dopamine, which reduce the stress hormones in the body such as cortisol and nor-epinephrine.

- Massage produces a 'relaxation response". An involuntary response in which heart rate and breathing slow, stress hormones decrease, serotonin is released, and muscle relax. As discussed earlier, it is the vagus nerve that slows heart rate and decreases blood pressure.

- Massage decreases pain by disturbing signals to the brain and helping to "close the pain gate." It reduces Substance P, which acts as a neurotransmitter altering cellular signaling pathways and decreasing sensitivity to pain.

- Massage reduces inflammation in the body by improving circulation and removing fluid build-up. Massage releases cytokines known as Interleukin- 4(IL4) and Interleukin 10(IL10), which have anti-inflammatory effects.

- Massage reduces stress by decreasing muscle tension and increasing body temperature, which promotes relaxation. It also reduces ACTH (adenocorticotropic hormone), which stimulates cortisol, a stress hormone.

- Massage increases available level of serotonin, which has positive effects on emotion and thought.

- Massage, using moderate pressure, increases theta brain waves, which accompany relaxation.

- Massage enhances sleep by releasing serotonin, which is derived from the amino acid tryptophan. Serotonin is converted to melatonin in the brain, which influences the sleep stage of an individual's circadian rhythm.

- Massage boosts our immune system by flushing out toxins and increasing circulation and lymphatic flow. It also works on the immune system by increasing natural killer cells (an immune cell), which are the front lines of our immune system and kill viral infected cells.

- Massage boosts the lymphatic system, stimulating circulation and the removal of metabolic wastes generated in the body.

- Massage promotes release of histamine, a neurotransmitter, that increases the permeability of blood vessels, increasing vasodilation. Vasodilation, which causes blood vessels to widen and become closer to the skin, increases relaxation, decreases pain, and can help with preparing the body for exercise or competition.

These are just some of the many mechanisms and benefits massage brings.

THE BODY REMEMBERS AND SPEAKS ITS MIND

How Emotional Trauma Manifests in the Body

Albert Einstein has speculated that rational science reveals only the external experience of some deeper reality. Understanding how emotions and trauma get trapped in the body is extremely valuable. As a hands-on practitioner, I believe it is more critical than ever to Understand not only how these get trapped, but to be able to know how they can be released with bodywork. Emotions are mental stimuli, a complex reaction pattern involving experimental behavior and physiological elements (UWA, Psychology and Counseling News).

Often confused with feelings and mood, emotions are physiological states and should not be interchanged with feelings and mood. Feelings arise from an emotional experience, and mood is a shorter-lived emotional state of usually low intensity; both lack stimuli and have no clear starting point. For example, when we experience the emotion fear, our heart beats faster, and we may sweat, shake, or freeze up. This is a physiological response and is the result of the autonomic nervous system's reaction to the emotion that was experienced. There can also be a healthy counterpart to emotions. Fear may paralyze some, while for others it provides the stimulus and motivation to move to higher and deeper levels of awareness and achievement. All emotions are inevitable and normal when they arise in daily life. They only become problematic when they're excessive, prolonged, or both. When traumatic experiences aren't consciously dealt with they can result in chronic fear, stress, and even occurrences of PTSD.

Trauma is considered anything that keeps us locked in physical, emotional, behavioral, or mental habit. When trauma occurs, our bodies activate a protective mechanism. A stressor that is too much for a person to handle overloads the nervous system, stopping the trauma from processing. This overloads and halts the body in its instinctive fight/ flight/freeze response, causing the traumatic energy to be stored in the surrounding muscles, organs, and connective tissue. Whenever we store trauma in our tissue, our brain disconnects from that part of the body to block the experience, preventing the recall of the traumatic memory. Any area of our body that our brain is disconnected from won't be able to stay healthy and heal (Barnes, JF). As Peter Levine so effectively states, "No animal, not even the human has conscious control over whether or not it freezes in response to threat."

This state of immobility is beyond conscious control and becomes a vicious cycle maintaining physiological high levels of activity of both the parasympathetic and sympathetic nervous systems (Barnes, JF). The body is a map of every experience we ever had. Any area of our body that our brain is disconnected from won't be able to stay healthy and heal unless we properly address it.

UNLOCKING THE CAGE USING EASTERN & WESTERN MODALITIES

Certain bodywork styles effectively reduce stress and tension, allowing release as well as function to reconnect the brain with the stored trauma. As I mentioned earlier, my first teachings of massage and understanding of the human body were of Eastern tradition. The first bodywork I ever learned was in Thailand, studying Traditional Thai Massage at Wat Pho (The Temple of the Reclining Buddha) in Bangkok, continuing on with advanced training in Medical Thai massage on the magical island of Kho Phan Ghan with my teacher Nipha Sankhawai. It is through these teachings that I first came to understand Eastern tradition of a whole-body approach through bodywork.

Thai Massage

The basic principles of Thai massage ensure the flow of energy through the energy channels (meridians)m improving blood circulation throughout the body. Thai massage can benefit almost every organ in the body.

For example, a headache is not just in the head according to Eastern medicine, nor is it merely a pain or something to be stopped with regards to its origin, and never, ever treated on the basis of someone else's headache. Rather, it is an obstruction of qi (energy) that can be related to one's lifestyle. Treatment might include work on other areas like the legs and arms as well as or instead of the head, and may bring more lasting and positive changes that will attempt to block the superficial systems. Eastern philosophy regards everything as mutually conditioned rising together.

Shiatsu

Shiatsu is a holistic discipline developed in Japan. This comprehensive treatment system is based on the same concepts and roots with Chinese Acupuncture and Traditional Chinese Medicine (TCM). According to this theory, the human body and its internal organs function with the power and influence of Qi (energy). Shiatsu restores this balance of energy in our body, bringing harmony between these aspects of our life. It is a whole-body approach treatment. Although Shiatsu literally means "finger pressure," the essence of Shiatsu is communication through rhythmic touch. The treatment also uses stretching and is focused mainly along specific channels (meridians) from where the body Qi (energy) passes through. Using the bladder/kidney meridian as an example will give you a glimpse of how it works.

In Traditional Chinese medicine, the bladder is one of the six yang organs that are paired with the kidney, one of the six yin organs. Yin organs store vital substances (such as Qi, blood, yin and yang), whereas the yang organs are more active and have a function of constantly filling and emptying. The bladder is a yang organ whose main physiological function is storing and excreting the urinary waste fluids passed down from the kidneys. For this to happen, the bladder uses Qi (energy) and heat from its paired yin organ, the kidney. Therefore, the bladder system in Traditional Chinese Medicine has far more influence in the body than over just fluid transformation and excretion. And as an energy system, the bladder channel is initially related to the autonomic nervous system. This is because the bladder meridian (the longest meridian channel) runs along the back of the body from the eyes to the little toe, with two parallel branches flowing along each side of the spine. These 4 branches of the bladder meridian directly influence the sympathetic and parasympathetic trunks of the autonomous nervous system, which regulates our fight or flight response and in turn all the body's basic vital functions. I particularly pay attention to the two branches of the meridian that run along both sides of the spine. This is where the nerves emerge from the spine to enervate the body.

Massage to the bladder meridian has the palpable effect of relieving headaches and back pain, and can be helpful when one has eye pain, lack of bladder control, or a cold virus. Working this meridian not only has physiological effects; there also can be an emotional response. In Traditional Chinese medicine there is an emotion connected to the organs.

The emotion associated with the kidneys and bladder is fear. So, if the bladder meridian is not regulating, you can be experiencing an emotional/psychological response as well. As mentioned earlier, massaging this channel directly stimulates the parasympathetic nervous system and encourages one to feel more relaxed and peaceful. As you can see, releasing tension in the back and stimulating the bladder meridian will automatically release the stored psychic tension, resolving many physical and psychological problems.

Mayan Abdominal Massage

Another of my favorite, profound techniques that I had the privilege of studying in Guatemala is Mayan Abdominal Massage, a technique using mostly external massage to the abdomen and pelvis. My trainings were taught by Dona Dominga, a Kakchiquel midwife from the San Marcos La Laguna region of Guatemala.

The Mayans believe that many human emotions are stored in the abdomen. They aren't alone in that belief, as many cultures focus on the abdomen as a source of healing and power. In addition to physically releasing deep tension and refreshing the blood flow to muscles and organs, Mayan abdominal massage also reopens blocked energy paths and can release blocked Qi, life force as they call it, that has accumulated due to pent-up emotions (Avrigo, R.). This massage can be done on men, children and women. In women it is used specifically to help the uterus contract back to its adequate place after birth. After performing Mayan abdominal massage, a long woven fabric (commonly called a faja) is tied around the abdomen to help support the work, keeping the heart down (Mayans believe the heart is in the stomach) while at the same time supporting the body to directly affect the lower back. This a deep work acting as an energetic surging on the body, emotionally and physically. Allowing and supporting the release is part of the healing process.

Myofascial Release & Unwinding

With regards to emotional and physical trauma, the most profound teachings I had were taught to me in the West through "The John F. Barnes Myofascial Release Approach," taught by Barnes himself. John Barnes is a trained physical therapist who studied manipulative procedures from Dr. James Mennell, one of the forefathers of massage, mentioned earlier in my section on the history of massage. Barnes then went on to conceptualize his own theory of treatment. It was in the John Barnes approach that I learned extensively about the connective tissue system as well as soft tissue mobilization as a means to relieve pain and restore function. It focuses primarily on the fascial system.

Fascia is an incredible tough connective tissue that spreads throughout the body like a spider web from head to foot without interruption. Fascia supports, protects, envelops, and becomes part of the muscles, nerves, organs, and blood vessels, from the largest structures right down to the cellular level. When all is well, the body functions in harmony. However, when injuries occur, the fascia has the ability to reorganize along the lines of tension imposed on the body. Physical trauma from direct injury or accidents can cause the fascia to tighten down in an involuntary attempt to protect the body from further harm. As an injury remains unresolved, the reorganization of the fascia becomes more pronounced. Fascial strains slowly tighten, causing the body to lose its normal ability to act and react to its environment. It has been estimated that myofascial restrictions can create a tensile strength of up to approximately 2,000 pounds per square inch (Katake, K.). This enormous and excessive pressure of the myofascial restrictions on pain- sensitive structures can produce many of the pains, headaches, and undesirable symptoms that many people suffer. Most of these go undiagnosed because our standard medical tests (X-rays, CAT scans, EMG) do not show fascial restrictions (Barnes, JF.).

Patients with fascial restrictions are usually told that nothing is wrong with them or that their condition is arthritis and in some cases psychosomatic. Sometimes the patient is never even touched. Touching patients with skilled hands can be one of the most potent ways of locating fascial restrictions and effecting positive change. Touching through massage, movement therapy, or refined touch of myofascial release helps to enhance function and movement of every structure in the body. Myofascial release helps remove the pressure caused by restricted fascia, easing symptoms of pain, headaches, spasm, and fibromyalgia, and restoring range of motion. Myofascial release is a whole-body approach designed to rectify the fascial restrictions that caused the effect or symptom. While having been trained in all of John Barnes' myofascial release courses, it wasn't until his myofascial unwinding course that I experienced the most profound experience connecting mind and body releasing both state that before taking any of the myofascial courses, although having been trained in many Eastern whole-body approaches, I was working in a more traditional medical rehabilitation center in stroke and brain trauma, using more linear thinking and sometimes being skeptical of what might be known as esoteric or "energy" work.

The best way for me to describe myofascial unwinding is the spontaneous movement of the body via the mind in response to the therapist's touch. During fascial unwinding, the therapist stimulates mechanoreceptors in the fascia by applying gentle touch and stretching. The client responds with spontaneous bending, rotating, and twisting of the upper or lower limbs or of the whole body in either a rhythmic or a chaotic pattern. Despite how mystical this sounds, its results are effective and profound.

My first experience as a student in myofascial unwinding took place in a hotel's ballroom at one of Barnes' seminars. When he first demonstrated the technique on the stage, using one of the students as his model, I was stunned, shocked, and overwhelmed. This was exactly the type of "energy" work I steered clear of for many years. The emotional energy coming forth in the room was disturbing and at first disruptive. In the darkness of the room I became deeply fixated while working as the giver, then I was jolted by someone screaming, moaning, choking, or doing all three at once. I wondered to myself, "Am I experiencing an exorcism?," I was beginning to get scared and leery of this technique. After performing the unwinding on my partner, I was becoming more and more skeptical. Some of the people sitting around me were stressed to the point of wanting to escape. We looked at each other in disbelief, at the same time consoling and supporting each other.

It was now my turn to be the receiver. I was steadfast in my thinking that none of this emotional release would ever happen to me. As I lay on the table, my practitioner began with touch to my head and neck. Within moments, I suddenly felt my eyes start to flutter, my head began to roll from side to side, and heat rushed to my throat, at which point my practitioner placed her hands on my throat. I began to cough and choke. The throat has always been a spot I have weakness in. Growing up as a very shy girl, I often felt I didn't have a voice. There were master practitioners walking around and one approached my table and begin to assist my practitioner, repeating over and over, "let it go, scream, yell, let your voice be heard." In my head I kept thinking, "this can't be happening to ME." My left arm began to circle around receptively (I had a previous injury to my left shoulder).

Before I knew it I was thrashing about the table, proceeding to go into a complete headstand (one of my greatest fears in yoga) and here I was on a soft massage table actually doing one. I then continued to contour my body in all shapes and forms I never thought possible, continuing until I was slithering off the massage table to the floor, the entire time being guided by two practitioners. Oddly enough, I felt completely safe. When I completed my "unwinding" I could feel a sense of peace, as if 1000 pounds had been lifted off me. A few years earlier, I experienced an allergic reaction to an antibiotic resulting in severe neuropathy throughout my entire body. I had been dealing with the pain trauma for many years, explaining my intense response to the unwinding.

This may sound extremely esoteric to some. To better explain it, studies show that during long periods of trauma, people make indelible imprints of experience that have high levels of emotional content. The body can hold information below the conscious level, as a protective mechanism, so that memories become dissociated. The memories are state- or position-dependent and can therefore be retrieved when the person is in a particular state or position (Rossi, et al,16). It has been demonstrated consistently that when a myofascial release takes the tissue to a significant position, or when myofascial unwinding allows a body part to assume a significant position, the tissue not only changes and improves, but memories and associated emotional states also rise to the conscious level. The therapist acts as a facilitator, following the body's inherent motion (Barnes, JF).

In the days to come during the seminar, I looked around the room and I could see the difference in the faces and body language of all the students. I noticed the ones who did the most unwinding were walking taller, their faces glowed, shoulders were relaxed, and most important their hearts were open to everyone around them. This work is powerful. I continue to practice it today on clients and have seen incredible physical and emotional releases. I have seen patients relive car accidents, athletes go into the exact position they were injured in, and many suffering from fibromyalgia get an enormous sense of relief. The list goes on. It's extremely gratifying to see clients relieved from pain and emotions they were holding for years, with most of them having tried numerous modalities that failed to address the pain or injury. My own testimonial as well as the experiences of my many clients speaks to this incredible healing through myofascial unwinding.

I am grateful to all to my clients and patients who have taught me in my path. And I am honored to have had the privilege of learning this wonderful technique from John Barnes. He has not only taught me but shown me that "the body keeps the score." These techniques I have described are just a few examples of whole-body system approaches.

KEEPING IN TOUCH WITH YOURSELF

It is of utmost importance to not only listen and get to know your body, but to take time to receive treatment. If treatment is not an option, teaching ourselves the tools to meet our needs can be as beneficial. To restore your body and dissolve stored blocked emotions, first allow yourself to feel them. One of the best ways to get rid of muscle tension is to actively feel and let go of emotions as they come. Feeling the emotions might involve any form of catharsis like running, dancing, deep belly breathing, screaming or crying. This is called emotional regulation, which is our ability to cope with stress in a flexible, tolerant, and adaptive way.

Our attitude matters, and it is important we come from a place of nonjudgment. When we consider our emotions as something bad or wrong, we actually deepen our suffering and solidify the tensions within our bodies. Instead, surrender to each emotion. Become aware of yourself. Our deepest challenge is to recognize the emotion and feel it in our body. This is where mindfulness is helpful. Notice what is happening, and accept and feel it fully without judging. Be gentle and kind with yourself. This might sound simple, but it's profound. Muscle tension tends to add to our inner voices, which cause us even more tension. Find a trained practitioner and receive bodywork. If this is not an option, self- massage, meditation, and breathing techniques are all extremely beneficial. While self- massage caters to our physical state, it can also unwittingly play a role in our mental state. Self-care helps us learn to identify and care for our physical and emotional needs.

Self-Massage Techniques

- Take time to do self-massage in a relaxing setting. Dimmig lights, lighting candles, or even going in nature can help promote more relaxation.

- Using aromatherapy is extremely beneficial. Your brain responds to smell and aromas. Essential oils added to a cream or a base oil like almond oil complement touch. Never apply essential oils directly to skin. Besides smelling, good essential oils also stimulate specific brain action.

- Grapefruit oil can promote release of endorphins, neurotransmitters that act as natural pain killers.

- Marjoram oil can boost your levels of serotonin, helping you feel calm.

- Sandalwood oil releases both dopamine and serotonin.

- Lavender, one of the more familiar oils, is known to promote relaxation and sleep.

- Ylang-ylang, a tropical plant native to India, Indonesia, and the Philippines, triggers the release of the "feel good" endorphins and serotonin.

When practicing self-massage techniques, it is more beneficial to use less physical pressure. When too much pressure is applied, our bodies naturally fight the pain by contracting our muscles, making the massage harder to enjoy. We have tightness in our body due to overuse, stress, and anxiety. Stress and anxiety are more mental responses, so keeping the pressure light is best for these. You can use a deeper pressure for soreness or injuries.

Shoulders & Neck

These always comprise an area of muscle tension and stress. Begin with one side of your shoulders at a time, hooking your fingers over the trapezius muscle (your bulky shoulder muscle that is easily palpated) and knead with your fingers, being sure to focus and keep pressure on areas of increased muscle tension. To create deeper depth, lower your ear to the opposite shoulder to stretch the trapezius muscles as you continue to massage the area.

Abdominal Massage

Abdominal massage can ease bloating and encourage waste to be dispersed. Use both hands to stroke the stomach, going in a circular motion including the sides of the waist. Lastly, stroke the abdomen up the right hand side, across the top and down the left hand side. This is the pathway of the colon. Remember that the abdomen can be a place where emotions get stored. Massaging this area can release anything that is blocked.

Reflexology

Reflexology, a type of massage using pressure to the feet, is based on a theory that areas of the feet are related to certain organs and body systems throughout the body.

• **Diaphragm Reflex** - located along the entire mid foot. Using your thumb, work across the middle of the foot 3 times. Working this point helps to release tension held in the entire body.

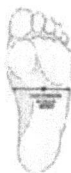

• **Pituitary Reflex** - Using your thumb, press and circle the middle of the big toe for a few seconds. The pituitary gland is found at the base of the brain and is often referred to as "the master gland" of the body. This gland produces many hormones and is responsible for releasing hormones that stimulate the adrenal glands, the thyroid gland, the ovaries, and the testes. Repeat at least 3 times.

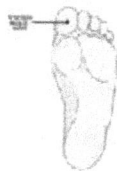

• **Spinal reflexes** - Using the thumb, press and circle down the side of the foot, starting from the big toe down towards the heel. Next, press and move across from the heel to the ankle to the big toes along the side of the foot. Repeat at least 3 times.

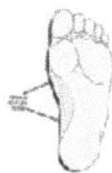

Shiatsu/Acupressure

The acupoint LI 20, English name Welcome Fragrance and Pinyin name Ying Xiang, is a very powerful point to treat all kinds of conditions related to the nose and sinuses. With so many suffering from allergies, this is a wonderful point to work. In Traditional Chinese Medicine the large intestine is paired with the lungs (yin and yang). Both of these organs represent our ability to be "open" or taking in, and "letting go" or releasing. In the body, their channel-pathways can be used to create space in congested areas. This point can be located at the level with the midpoint of the lateral border alanasi (also known as the side of the nostril). It lies right above the largest sinus pocket in our head and is the last point on the large intestine meridian. You may wonder why a large intestine point is on the face. The concept of "letting go" on the face is analogous to that of our bowel function: both are a physiological process of releasing what no longer is needed to nourish our body. When we experience cold symptoms such as sinusitis, this is also a form of releasing accumulation, a clearing out of what does not serve the body. By pressing into this area we can improve fluid circulation and open the airway for better breathing, releasing any pressure you may have in this area. It is a good point to use when suffering from rhinitis, sinusitis, acne, abscesses of the mouth, and toothache, to name a few.

ACUPOINT: LI20

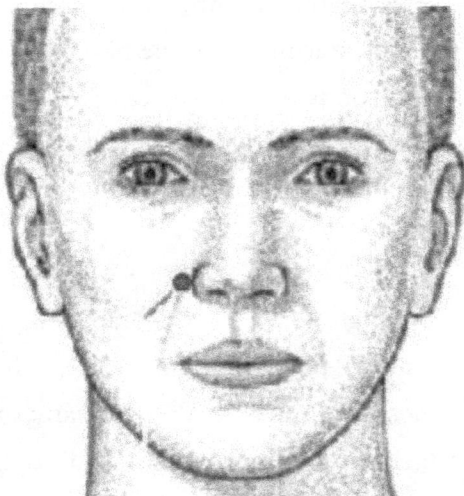

Thai Massage Stretch

A beneficial pose in Thai massage is Supine Spinal Twist. Start by lying flat on your back. The first thing to do is bring one leg across the body, slowly rotating your body in the opposite direction. Let your gaze follow, then take a moment to pause and breathe while holding the position.

The many benefits of Supine Spinal Twist include quieting the nervous system, and stretching the gluteals, external obliques, and abdominal muscles. Internal organs are toned during abdominal stretching. Supine Spinal Twist is also conducive to digestion and relieves constipation. Tension in the back is also relieved and fatigue is alleviated. In general, twists allow more nourishment to reach the roots of the spinal nerves, and this has a positive effect on the sympathetic nervous system. There are some contraindications that should be noted with Supine Spinal Twist. These include pregnancy, spinal operations, herniated discs, degenerative disc diseases, and sciatica.

~ ~ ~ ~ ~ ~ ~

Most important to understand is that your biology, experiences, environment, careers, and emotional states are your own and unique to you alone. These are all connected to who you are and what manifests within you. In listening to your mind, body, and spirit you can best determine what makes you feel nourished, what you need and how you can adapt and care for yourself. This is the first step to apply, which can be more profound than any application or technique.

It is then that you will be able to comprehend your structural relationships, which can assist you to seek a practitioner with these needs in mind. Find the right person or modality that fits your unique being. A qualified and experienced practitioner will guide you in your journey to heal from pain restrictions, injuries, trauma, anxiety, or whatever it is you may be experiencing, but remember it is your journey and you are your best guide. It may never be as simple as one modality or treatment, and it may be as simple or not so simple as learning to breathe, relax, or calm your mind and body. You and only you will be able to know what is right and how you can expand on it. Life is a process of multiple states we encounter. Embracing each one is part of the journey. It is when we remain in a state that restrictions and holding patterns are created.

Be present, expand, and dare to blossom!

WORKS CITED

Avrigo R., Epstein N. Rainforest Home Remedies: The Maya Way to Heal Your Body & Replenish Your Soul 2001)

Barnes , JF. Myofascial Release: The Search for Excellence. Philadelphia: Rehabilitation Sciences Inc. 1990)

Carlson, M. & Earles F. (1997) Psychological and neuroendocrinological msequel of our social deprivation in institutionalized children in Romania.

Engel G. The Need for a new medical mode: a challenge for Biomedicine Science.1977; 196:129-136

Field, Tiffany M., et al (1986) "Tactile/Kinesthetic Stimulation Effects on Pre-term Neonatals Pediatics. 77(5): 654-658)

-------- (1999), Pre schoolers in America are Touched less and more aggressive than pre-schoolers in France, Early Development and Care, 151:1, 11-17.

-------- Massage Therapy Research (1st edi.) Edinburgh: Elsevier Churchill Livingston, 2006

Katake, K.1961: The strength for tension and bursting of human fascia. J. Kyoto Med. Univ. 69:484-488.

Kurtz R. Body centered psychotherapy: the Hakomi therapy, Ashland, OR: Author of the Hakomi Institute, 1988

Linden, D. (2015) The Power of Touch, The New Yorker

Ni, Maoshing, Ph. D., The Yellow Emperor's Classic of Medicine: A New Translation of the Neijing Suwen with Commentary. 1995.

Rossi, E.L.(1987) From mind to molecule. A state-dependent memory, learning and behavior theory of mind-body healing. Advances, 4(2). 46-60 "The Science of Emotion Exploring the Basics of Emotional Psychology," Psychology and Counseling News. UAW Online, June 27, 2019. https://online.uwa.edu/news/emotional-psychology/

CHAPTER X

My Eastern Paths to Healing
Sharon Dominguez

We have heard the poets say it and the astrophysicists alike: we are nature. We are the universe. We are both creation and creators, one with the source of life. We are the sun and the stars and the earth we walk upon. Our luminous beings are made up of the same elements that make up the entire existence of the cosmos. We are governed by electromagnetism and the laws of nature. Yin and Yang. This is who we are as individual beings and collectively as a whole.

How connected we are to these truths directly affects the quality of our human experience. When we live in accordance to the laws of nature, we are in a state of balance. Balance is health, the alignment of body, mind and spirit. Our energy is fluid like a river. Perhaps you have had the experience of being in the flow. You have seen athletes in the zone, masterful artists who have taken your breath away. The confluence of body, mind, and spirit working in concert with each other is the balance of life itself. Balance also occurs as we are harmonious with nature. Like a tree in the spring, when buds form, soon to flower and bloom, such is replicating in our own bodies too. Our energy in the beginning of spring is beginning to expand. By summer, like the sun, our life energy is its most expansive. By the autumn, we enter the gathering phase, not unlike the harvest to prepare for winter, where we contain stored fuel. This is the cycle of the seasons as well as the cycle of our body. We are created to follow nature.

Sickness, on the other hand, happens when we break that natural cycle. When a patient comes into my office, chances are, their systems are off cycle, even compromised. Like those of many holistic professionals, my services are often sought after exhausting other more mainstream avenues. Perhaps patients have a sinking winter pulse in the middle of summer, indicating a cold or kidney/bladder issues. They might be suffering from symptoms like lethargy, frequent urination, thirst, or back pain. Together, we begin the process of restoring their system to harmonize once again with the laws of nature.

Balance—I wish it sounded sexier. If only we could choose the red pill or the blue pill. Beginning with formulating a diagnosis, I am confronted more often than not with what I describe as a knotted chain that needs to be unraveled. Piece by piece, we undo the blocks created by a myriad of causes, from poor diet, physical injury, emotional and psychological imbalances, trauma, insomnia, viruses, and pathogens, to genetic predispositions. While Western medicine focuses on treating illness, holistic medicine addresses health and wellness in a biopsychosocial approach. We treat the cause of the imbalance where mainstream medicine focuses on the treating the effects. Each treatment is a building block to remove old patterns and blockages in order to restore the system to its full potential.

Eastern medicine is a road map. In the body, there are points that form part of a meridian, which is a pathway of energy. We refer to this energy as Qi or Ki. Every meridian relates to the function of an organ in the body and its system. Every system correlates with the elements of nature. As we return to health, we are restoring all of nature. When we live in accordance to nature, we are repairing nature itself and protecting ourselves from pathogenic sickness. I can't properly articulate the wonder I experienced hearing this for the first time, that there is a harmony in the universe which expresses itself in the form of sound, frequency, energy, electromagnetism, light—and that our enlightened ancients, connected to the source of life, were able to preserve in detail an innate understanding of the laws of life and to preserve a detailed medicine that we still use today, a medicine that has more relevance as people seek to heal.

Life, as I knew it as a child, couldn't have been farther from the life the ancients described. My story is a common one you hear all the time, of a practitioner whose interest in healing was sparked by her own health challenges. When I was a child, I suffered from ongoing pain, doubled over from pain, and staying home from school kinds of digestive issues.

This often led to my attraction to foods which only increased my discomfort. In a continuous spiral, I resorted to strong laxatives, on which I became dependent before I was 13. On my own, I would put myself on severe diets, hoping that would make me feel better. Even though I was athletic, I was dysmorphic, my body a source of struggle and pain. Not a single doctor could diagnose me, neither my pediatrician nor my parents' primary doctor—or the cadre of specialists whose tests and diets often made things worse. During one of those times, when I was eleven, I decided to eat only sugary fruit yogurt for breakfast, lunch, and dinner: mono-eating, what I now know is a sure sign that the system is off. There were the protein powders given to me by a specialist, a famous doctor who inaccurately diagnosed me with hypoglycemia, low blood sugar. His dietary guide of an all-protein diet made me even sicker and more sluggish. There was the summer I ate only mixed salad. I was intolerably hungry, but afraid to eat.

My teenage years were marked by cystic acne and an overactive, unbalanced hormonal system. I rarely felt good. My emotional state

237

was so out of whack, I often medicated with recreational drugs. Doctors gave me ongoing antibiotic therapy to help my skin. My digestive system worsened. I no longer remembered what feeling good, or well, was like. I was anxious and couldn't sleep. Then came the muscle relaxers for a nervous stomach.

Nobody could correctly diagnose me. However, I had an inkling that something was missing. When I was around 12, I found a book on the street called The Herb Book, by John Lust, a book on herbs from the Northern Hemisphere called the most complete catalog of "miracle plants" ever published. I was riveted and dog- eared all the pages. The book contained recipes for concoctions and teas to heal various conditions, including infusions for my digestive woes, but I had no idea where to find the herbs. Where was Google when I needed it?

One day, I entered a store that sold hippie products like lava lamps, rock and roll posters, candles, and silver jewelry. I found packets of Belladonna and Damiana, which I excitedly bought having seen their names in The Herb Book. I took them home, but when I read that Belladonna was poisonous if not dosed properly and Damiana was an aphrodisiac, I left them untouched. I was a little kid and I didn't want to accidentally poison myself, nor was I ready to have sex. Through the years, I accumulated books on metaphysics, herbs, tarot, hand analysis, crystals. I had a nagging sense that there was something more to life, but it was just not yet revealed to me.

On a trip to Chiapas, Mexico, when I was 17 years old, I picked up a book on medicine of the Ancient Maya at the library of Casa Na Bolom, an inn and sanctuary created by anthropologist Frans Blum and his wife Gertrude. I read through the healing methods of the local shamans, the extensive knowledge of ethnobotany, the connection to the divine life force and the cycles of nature, and even some dangerous remedies including putting feces on your head, as a last resort to ward off death (not to worry, I have never prescribed that in my practice!). The book described the animal spirits, the power of the Nahuatl (the jaguar), and all the different deities. For me it was a mix of plant wisdom and the spirit world, of which I had zero understanding. I was surprised how comprehensive the system was for something that was recorded so many hundreds of years ago.

Everything changed for me during my college years. In my freshman year, my faculty advisor, a professor of Eastern and Indian studies, took 15 of us to see Swami Jiddu Krishnamurti. He was seated on the floor on a large stage at an outdoor arena, talking about life to an enthusiastic crowd of devotees. I think I might've fallen asleep, lulled by the drone of his voice and my resistance. However, listening to him was also a catalyst for a journey that has never ended: the world of spirit and the search for the meaning of life. By my senior year of college, I was hoping to embark on a career as a Classical musician; I didn't know it then, but in the summer of 1984 I attended a weekend workshop that was going to change the course of my life.

His name was Sensei Masahilo M Nakazono, the founder of a school in Santa Fe, New Mexico called the Kototama Institute. There, he and his two sons were training students to be doctors of an esoteric form of Eastern Medicine called Inochi, based on the Kototama Principle, the sounds according to Shinto that make up our entire existence. We spent that weekend in August, 1984 learning about the governing laws of life, energy frequencies, sounds, nature, and health. He talked about universal truths as told by the ancestors. I cried for days, with an inner knowing, like coming home.

That week, I also met Dr. Neal, a naturopath who would start me on my personal journey to healing. It was determined that I had, among other things, an overgrowth of yeast in my system, the prime environment for pathogenic bacteria to thrive. The cause? Overuse of antibiotics. I had almost no healthy intestinal flora. Additionally, my diet was making it worse. He muscle-tested me, which led to dietary changes, such as the removal of yeast, wheat, sugar, meat, dairy, caffeine, alcohol, nightshades, vinegar, etc. He replaced them with whole grains, fruit and vegetables, chicken, fish, legumes, oils. I added therapeutic levels of probiotics, homeopathic remedies, exercise and other supplements to support holistic healing from within. I followed the regimen religiously and it paid off, finally knowing what it was like to feel good, and well. My mind was clear, my energy was vibrant, my digestive system became regular. I slept well, and my body both felt and looked fit. My outlook on life improved as I felt a sense of gratitude and well-being. I wanted everyone to feel this way, to know what it was like to be integrated.

In 1985, after a year in Italy amid a failing marriage, playing and teaching music, studying natural medicine from anyone who'd teach me, metaphysical workshops, and diminished health from stress, Italian food, and an abundance of despair, I returned to New York to pursue my Master's degree in music at NYU. Meanwhile, I was invited to attend a two-week workshop on healing with Inochi Medicine by Nakazono's son Jei, exactly a year after I attended his dad's seminar. I dove in. Jei handed out his translation of The Yellow Emperor, The Lost Books Of The Su Wen. It further opened my eyes to a holistic world, where everything turned out to be part of the laws of nature. Its prologue says:

> The ancients thought that there were five indispensable qualities for living. These are Wood, Fire, Earth, Metal and Water,

and they are otherwise known as the five phases. They each possess different characteristics, and all phenomena and substances within the universe belong to one of these five phases. The idea which has developed into the five-phase theory is that all phenomena and substances in the universe are the products of the movement and mutation of these five phases. The five-phase theory, as described in the Neijing, is a philosophical theory of medical practice in ancient China. This theory has served as the guiding ideology and methodology of physiology, pathology, clinical diagnosis and treatment. The characteristics of each phase in this theory have been derived from the observations of countless generations over the millennia, and they are reflected in clinical experiences (Ni).

In addition to The Yellow Emperor, Jei handed us each a five elementchart. It blew my mind how everything in the universe could be synthesized into five categories. There were five sounds, five directions, five yin organs, five yang organs, five elements, five emotions, five senses, five tastes, five virtues, the list was endless, showing how our entire world belonged within the system like a whole, interconnected circle of life. Everything exists within the flow of life; from matter, like a wooden table, to something subjective like worry. I learned about Yin and Yang, the laws of dualism. As defined by The Yellow Emperor, "The law of yin and yang is the natural order of the universe, the foundation of all things, mother of all changes, the root of life and death." I was taught that existence falls within the variabilities of darkness and light, and how yin and yang are both opposites, yet complementary, an interconnected circle from concentration to expansion and back, just like the seasons, the years, the months, the days, the hours, etc. There is even an Eastern Zodiac which also follows the universal cycle of Yin and Yang through twelve animal spirits. Anything that exists, I was taught, lives within the Taoist concept of time, space, and dimension. I learned what constitutes health, the harmony of the elements, and the disharmony that creates sickness.

During the two-week seminar, we practiced a form of handwork called Do-In, where we treated ourselves, using self-massage, and each other. My interest in bodywork and acupressure surprised me, as I was never that comfortable connecting to people through touch, but found myself feeling immense satisfaction at being both the patient and even more as the practitioner. More importantly, I started to get treated by Jei twice a week. He asked me many questions, the same ones I ask my patients to this day, to formulate a diagnosis. He read my pulses on my wrist and neck simultaneously to determine the root cause of my sickness. He told me that he was reading the state of my organs' systems and that he was going to use acupuncture to tonify and sedate my body's systems depending on what he deemed necessary. I so badly wanted to read what he was reading. My passion was ignited.

Through The Yellow Emperor, I also learned that these pulses have additional unique qualities which also correlate with an organ's system. For example, the heart pulse is a rapid pulse which has the sensation of a hook coming up and around on the finger, whereas the kidney pulse is a slow, sinking pulse. Liver pulse has the sensation of a tense violin string, and so on. There were also secondary and tertiary pulse qualities. 70 percent of treatment is diagnosis. I learned that to be integrated with nature, it is expected that you would have the pulse quality that corresponded to the season we were in. If you didn't, it was indicative of imbalance or even sickness.

In Eastern medicine, there are twelve primary meridians and eight extraordinary meridians. There are 361 main points and 48 extra points, The twelve primary meridians are pathways of energy (ki or Qi) of specific organs and viscera. The twelve meridians represent the flow of energy of the Liver, Gall Bladder, Heart, Small Intestine, Heart Constrictor (Pericardium), Triple Heater (the body's thermostat), Spleen, Stomach, Lung, Large Intestine, Kidney, and Bladder.

You read the condition of these systems on the pulses along the radial artery of the wrist. The Liver/Gall Bladder System relates season of spring, the phase of birth and consciousness. The Heart/Small Intestine System relates to summer, the growth and awareness. The Spleen/Stomach system is late summer (or the middle of each season), the phase of transformation and love. The Lung/Large Intestine system relates to the season of Fall, the phase of gathering and discernment or clarity. The Kidney/Bladder System relates to the season of winter, the phase of storing and wisdom.

Here is a short Five Element chart:

	Wood	Fire	Earth	Metal	Water
Orientation	East	South	Middle	West	North
Season	Spring	Summer	Late Summer	Autumn	Winter
Climate	Wind	Summer Heat	Dampness	Dryness	Cold
Cultivation	Germinate	Grow	Transform	Reap	Store
Yin Organ	Liver	Heart	Spleen	Lung	Kidney
Yang Organ	Gall Bladder	Small Intestine	Stomach	Large Intestine	Bladder
Orifice	Eye	Tongue	Mouth	Nose	Ear
Tissues	Tendons	Vessels	Muscles	Skin & Hair	Bones
Emotions	Anger	Joy	Pensiveness	Grief	Fear

Colour	Blue/Green	Red	Yellow	White	Black
Taste	Sour	Bitter	Sweet	Pungent	Salty
Voice	Shout	Laugh	Sing	Cry	Groan

The Meridians and their points are said to work with the nervous system. Our bodies look a lot like trees with a root system and branches.

Human body meridians

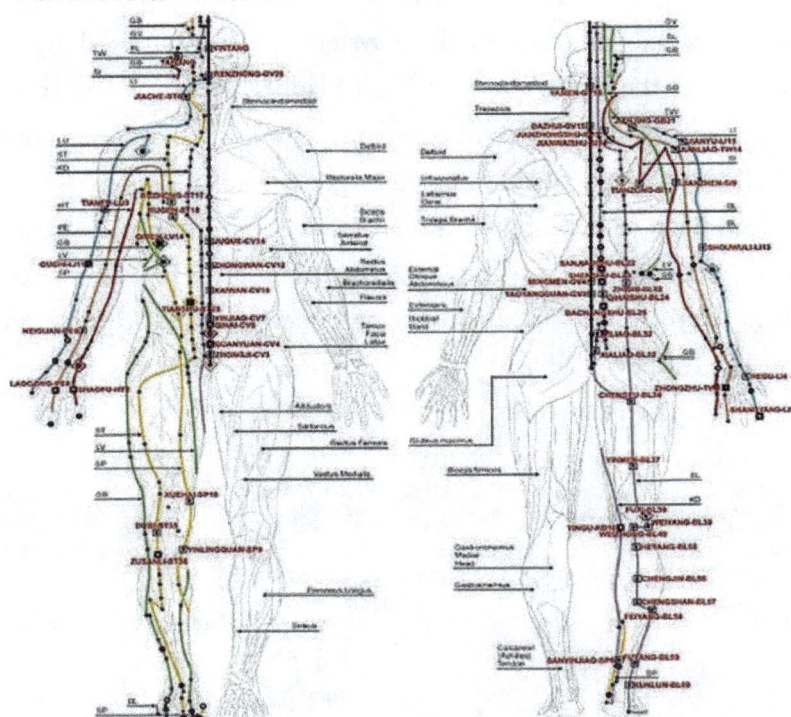

By the end of the two-week intensive, I was at a crossroads. Do I return to my marriage in Italy and my job teaching music, do I get my Masters at NYU, do I enter into the family business, or do I embark on a journey I never imagined for myself, studying to become a Doctor of Eastern medicine? At the time, there were so few people with careers herbology. Anyone and everyone tried to dissuade me. But, it was a friend of my parents' friend, an American doctor who spent time in China, who encouraged me to follow my heart. In January of 1986, my marriage and my music career were to become a distant memory. I showed up for my first class of Kototama Life Medicine and never looked back.

Eastern Medicine Explained

It is nearly impossible in a single chapter to explain Eastern Medicine, as vast as the universe itself. As I mentioned, everything that exists belongs to a circle of transformation. Life is change, so it follows that Eastern Medicine is a guide as to how to live by universal law, given perpetual change. According to The Yellow Emperor, the ancients had an innate intelligence for thousands of years, in which they naturally understood the flow of life. Chapter One of The Yellow Emperor is called "The Universal Truth," written within 2698-2598, BCE. Here is an excerpt that still resonates to me today as it did the first time I read it in September, 1985, nearly 37 years ago. The Yellow Emperor, Huang Di, is discussing medicine, lifestyle, and nutrition, along with Taoist cosmology with his ministers, Qi Bo and Lei Gong.

'I've heard that in the days of old everyone lived one hundred years without showing the usual signs of aging. In our time, however, people age prematurely, living only fifty years. Is this due to a change in the environment, or is it because people hav lost the correct way of life?' Qi Bo replied, 'In the past, people practiced the Tao, the Way of Life. They understood the prin-

245

ciple of balance, of yin and yang, as represented by the transformation of the energies of the universe. Thus, they formulated practices such as Dao-in, an exercise combining stretching, massaging, and breathing to promote energy flow, and meditation to help maintain and harmonize themselves with the universe. They ate a balanced diet at regular times, arose and retired at regular hours, avoided overstressing their bodies and minds, refrained from overindulgence of all kinds. They maintained well-being of body and mind; thus, it is not surprising that they lived over one hundred years. These days, people have changed their way of life. They drink wine as though it were water, indulge excessively in destructive activities, drain their jing—the body's essence that is stored in the kidneys—and deplete their qi. They do not know the secret of conserving their energy and vitality. Seeking emotional excitement and momentary pleasures, people disregard the natural rhythm and order of the universe.

They fail to regulate their lifestyle and diet, and sleep improperly. So it is not surprising that they look old at fifty and die soon after. The accomplished ones of ancient times advised people to guard themselves against zei feng (viruses and flus) disease-causing factors. On the mental level, one should remain calm and avoid excessive desires and fantasies, recognizing and maintaining the natural purity and clarity of the mind. When internal energies are able to circulate smoothly and endocand concentrated, illness and disease can be avoided. Previously, people led a calm and honest existence, detached from undue desire and ambition; they lived with an untainted conscience and without fear. They were active, but never depleted themselves. Because they lived simply, these individuals knew contentment, as reflected in their diet of basic but nourishing foods and attire that was appropriate to the season but never luxurious. Since they were happy with their position in life, they did not feel jealousy or greed. They had compassion for others and were helpful and honest, free from destructive habits. They remained unshakable and unswayed by temptations, and they were able to stay centered even when adversity arose. They treated others justly, regardless of their level of intelligence or social position.'

I was like, WOW! No two patients have the same pulses or diagnosis even if they both have the same illness. Nor are their treatment protocols the same. We are the sum of our parts, therefore unique. One patient's life experience will naturally differ from another's. One patient might drink alcohol every day, the other not. Lifestyle differences and genetic dispositions create different needs from the practitioner. Hence, while they could both have arthritis, one might be needled at the top edge of the small finger's fingernail, which begins the small intestine meridian, whereas another patient will receive moxibustion (burning hemp) along the large intestine meridian. This is radically different from allopathic medicine, which takes a one- size-fits-all approach to treating illness. It is the work of an Eastern doctor to peel away the layers, to undo the pathogenic flow of energy to one that is in tune with the cosmos.

In modern society, this has gotten rather complicated. We are pressured to follow life-depleting goals. Out of necessity, we follow the dollar bill, get swayed by illusory societal ideals. We spend countless moments away from the now, diving into our barrage of thoughts, feelings, and stressors. We waste energy trying to change others and expend priceless moments worrying about what other people think. This leaves us fragmented. Our bodies are often sedentary for hours at a time. It hurts me to see school-age kids sitting for their entire school day without an outlet for their life energy. No wonder we're sick. We are more polarized and divisive than ever, careening away from the natural order.

The ancients believed then that we need to find our way back to a simple, more authentic way of life, connected and interconnected. To regain or even retain health, we need to honor the seasons and our place within them. The Yellow Emperor writes, ""Health and well-being can be achieved only by remaining centered in spirit, guarding against the squandering of energy, promoting the constant flow of qi and blood, maintaining harmonious balance of yin and yang, adapting to the changing seasonal and yearly macrocosmic influences, and nourishing one's self preventively. This is the way to a long and happy life." There are plenty of examples of how we can weaken or strengthen the body. How well we follow the laws of nature in the spring can determine the state of our health in late summer. If we follow the guidelines as related to summer, we will be strong as we gather our energy in autumn to help in the winter months. That's how interdependent the cycles of the seasons are.

Humans have developed technologies to mitigate the effects of the bodies have acclimated to living less harshly in the elements. However, I do believe that in summer we need to be active and to sweat. It is how we remove toxins and avoid sickness later on. We have an inner thermostat that maintains the proper temperature within the body called the Triple Heater, that while it has adapted to modern ways, still benefits from the seasons that regulate us. As we are made up largely of fluids, we need to drink water throughout the year. However, we need to drink more water in the summertime when it's hot and there is danger of dehydration. Or even in autumn, the dry period. Constipation can be prevalent in winter due to the use of heating in our homes, which dehydrates the body.

While we need to drink water to counteract the dry heat, if we drink water that is too cold in the winter months it will hurt our kidneys. This can harm our physical stamina and life force. In winter, hot or room temperature liquids help us stay healthy. We will stay well if we abide by the common-sense rules. This includes doing what you can to preserve your life energy and not drain your ki.

Following the seasons and abiding by their rhythm is another way to protect ourselves. In winter, as the days are shorter, going to bed earlier will preserve our life force. Doing strenuous physical activity in extremely cold weather can weaken our kidney energy. Even the excess of sexual intercourse in winter can weaken our system. Overexerting is easier in the spring and summer months, when the life energy is at the most expansive.

We are what we eat!

When someone enters into my practice, the first order of business is to regulate the digestive system. There are too many illnesses to count either caused by or worsened by digestive irregularities or impairment. Inflammation in the gut alone is the cause of a myriad of sicknesses including autoimmune problems.

I cannot overstate the importance of not only eating according to the season, but internalizing that food is fuel or energy that nourishes us and keeps us alive, even helps us thrive. Many adverse health conditions can be mitigated or healed by diet. In a patient who is out of balance, I often use food as medicine, as what they are eating could be toxic, exacerbating their sickness. Not unlike what happened to me.

In the last 35 years, I have seen more and more patients with food allergies and sensitivities. Between overly processed, chemically enhanced food that is stripped of its properties, bodies have been compromised by their inability to break down and metabolize the food as it works its way through the digestive process. For example, simple sugar can cause havoc. Excess sweet taste causes an internal loosening which is the equivalent of an internal mudslide in our bodies. This can lead to symptoms like brain fog, fatigue, anxiety, aching, and stiff muscles, stomach pain, heartburn, even gout. In fact, too much of any one taste eaten repetitively can potentially make you sick. As all things, it all comes down to balance.

As a rule, a diet rich in nutrient-dense foods includes organic fruit and vegetables, locally sourced meat and fish, beans, whole grains, and fats. Nakazono used to recommend the 60/20/20 rule; 60 percent vegetables and fruit, 20 percent protein, and 20 percent whole grains.

Eating within a twelve-hour period and no later than 8pm, when the digestive energy is strong, is optimal. Of course, each person thrives on different things in any given moment. Food is fluid. Other food recommendations you would hear if you entered in my practice is to eat the colors of the rainbow. To incorporate all the tastes and their colors in your meals will nourish your organs and their systems. We need to strive for a balance of sour, bitter, sweet, hot (spicy), and salt, and the colors green, red, yellow or orange, white and black or purple to feed the liver, heart, spleen, lung and kidney systems, respectively.

There are five phases pertaining to our cycles. Spring is the birthing stage, when we can eat early foods like berries, cucumbers, asparagus, and sprouts, to name a few. Summer is the most bountiful, when we can eat the largest variety of seasonal fruits and vegetables. Spicy food is tolerated better during summer as it helps us sweat and dispel heat.

Late summer, still abundant, we have broccoli, string beans, corn, peaches, plums and nectarines. By fall, we enter into the gathering period, the time of the harvest; apples, pears, cabbage, squash, beets, and potatoes can be picked and stored for the long winter ahead. Winter, the storing periodm is a good time for root vegetables, hardy winter squash, warming foods, grains, soup, and stews. Along those lines, the Locavore movement recently took hold. The definition of locavore is "one who eats foods grown locally whenever possible." Coined on Earth Day in 2005, the movement was a way not only for people to eat healthfully and more nutritiously, but also for its positive impact on the environment as we move away from agribusiness to local individual farmers who tend to employ farming practices more sustainable for the planet, which includes avoiding harsh chemicals like pesticides and preservatives used to keep the produce alive during long trips. Lacavore is a natural way to align our diet to the seasons. Oftentimes, a clinician will offer dietary guidelines depending on the patient's diagnosis. This includes what foods and fluids will contribute to balancing the patient and which foods will continue the cycle of illness. Food can be medicine or it can be poison. Water is what we need to sustain ourselves, yet as in nature, too much water, with no place to go can be destructive. All of this can be complicated as people don't just eat for nutrition. I have discovered from my own experience that people have a challenging relationship with food: we also eat to placate an emotional need, which could be considered a form of self-soothing or other pathologies. It is often a part of our brain circuitry: food as reward, part of the Behavior Loop discussed in Chapter III (p. 50). On the other side, there is fear of food and the need to control. We have complicated a simple process naturally intended to use food as fuel.

Nakazono Sensei once told me that there was a time when we had the innate intelligence to know unequivocally what our body needed to thrive, including which tastes would make our body stay whole. This intelligence belonged to the hundred-year-olds mentioned in The Yellow Emperor. He said that acupuncture, which is the system of needling the patient, was considered drastic and extreme, not unlike Western surgery, by the people already in balance. In time, however, our ability to ascertain what would create or maintain balance waned. Today we are drawn by images in store windows, ads, cravings that override our healthy proclivities and our intuition of the steps we can take to regain balance. I remember when I was around five years old, there was a Twinkies commercial where every time a kid ate a Twinkie, he would grow tall. I believed it. In my house, growing up, you never found junk food. You have no idea how hard it was for me to convince my parents to buy me Twinkies so that I could grow as tall as the kids on the commercial. Twinkies came in a packet of two. Honestly, they were vile, way too sweet. But, look at the power of advertising! For immediate satisfaction, we can be swayed, which distances us from what we truly need to be well. In my practice, I have seen the effects of frozen coffee drinks as a direct cause of stomach issues. The mixture of caffeine as a stimulant, ice, dairy, and sugar is a quadruple whammy. How people drink these in winter is the pinnacle of disconnection from what the body needs. You might as well be drinking arsenic.

As far away as we have gone from living with the cycle of nature, I believe we can get it back through conscious retraining. For example, women who are pregnant get clear signals from the body as to what they need. When I was pregnant with my first child, I was eating my usual way back then, very cleanly, no refined sugar, no dairy, no red meat, no wheat or yeast. One day, on my way to work, having the urge

My Eastern Paths to Healing

to stop into a typical NY deli, I ordered an egg with cheese on a white seeded roll. I remember to this day how surprised I was by the clarity of this need, yet I knew decisively that it was what my body needed. Another evening, I made myself a huge a bowl of sautéed organic spinach with garlic. It was always my absolute favorite meal! I sat down to watch the Yankees game and put a bite of spinach in my mouth and I recoiled! The smell, the taste, I couldn't even put it in my mouth. I never heard from my body that clearly around food before. I ate a piece of organic steak instead. My body was happy. There was also a time when I was at a party seated next to a tray of dried fruit. Normally, I stayed away from dried fruit for two reasons: they are hard to digest and, more importantly, my mother never allowed junk food in the house, considering dried fruit as a treat. Needless to say, my association with dried fruit was that it was the ultimate booby prize. They were not Yodels! Anyway, that day, my eyes were drawn to a dried fig. Usually not a fig-fan, something told me I had to have it. I put one in my mouth and the flavor burst in such a way that reminded me of how I felt when I would guzzle water due to intense thirst after severe dehydration from strenuous activity. I ate five more. This went on for about a week, where I would eat about five dried organic figs and my body totally welcomed them. Then, one day, I went to eat one and the taste changed. My body no longer wanted them. Perhaps I needed the fiber, calcium or even potassium. When my system was satiated, I was done.

We can train our bodies to know what tastes we need in any given moment, bypassing the mind and our temporal desires and instead learning a process which requires intuition and sensitivity. Here is an exercise I recommend to patients, a quick mediation to sensitize them to the energy of the food as it relates to your system.

Food Awareness Meditation

Whatever food you are planning to eat, look at it, think of the taste of it, imagine the feeling in your mouth, your body. If it's something you can hold, feel its energy in your hand connect to your body. How does it make you feel? Do you have a feeling of opening or closing or nothing at all? Does it awaken your desire to eat it? Do you feel repelled? Maybe you feel nothing. That is okay too. This kind of awareness develops over time. Let's say that your body feels open to it when you sit down to eat it: can Take the time to chew. How does it feel? Are you attuned to the moment when your body signals that it has had enough? This is also something we can cultivate through mindful practice. As a rule, it is good to stop eating when you are 80 percent full. As it happens, as your body starts the digestive process, you will feel a hundred percent full within 10-20 minutes after eating. This is a re- education on the road to holistic health.

Connecting to the food we eat is a powerful process. Some people say grace as a way to show gratitude for the bounty. The Japanese clasp their hands together, bow slightly and say, "Itadakimasu," which is a way to thank the spirit of the organism for taking the precious gift of their life.

Using your senses is a helpful tool, like triage. Looking at the food with your eyes, tasting the food, feeling the consistency, hearing the chewing. We use our physical senses to both derive pleasure and receive its full nutritional value. For the food to have the most healing properties, it is best to chew until it's liquid before swallowing, thus getting all the nutrients out of the food and easing the digestive process.

Of course this is easier said than done. In my family, we scarfed our food, eating in a maniacal way—yet another factor in my years and years of digestive hell. One more thing I would like to emphasize where food is concerned is that food is also a form of divine pleasure. While I am not advocating for cheeseburgers or a slice of thin crust pizza, neither am I making any proclamations against them. In a perfect world, if you are in solid health, you should be able to enjoy whatever you want from time to time. As long as you eat slowly and with good spirit, no harm should come to you, and your body should inherently know how to restore itself. In fact, your conscious presence and state of being while eating is the last piece of the puzzle.

In 1992, when I was living, studying, and working in Santa Fe, New Mexico with Nakazono Sensei and his wife, I assisted him with an extensive guidebook for practitioners he was compiling on Kototama Life Therapy (no longer called Inochi Medicine). We tested hundreds of foods, products, and medicines to determine which systems they belonged to and, alternatively, which systems they could damage, so that we could use our knowledge of food and supplements to serve our patients.

We were conducting our experiments using applied kinesiology, a form of muscle testing, to see how the body reacted. One day, we performed an interesting experiment with a piece of chocolate and organic string beans. We muscle-tested the string bean and it came up healthful. Then, we muscle-tested the chocolate and it came up weak. Sensei put the string bean in my hand again and asked me to think angry thoughts; then, when he muscle-tested me, the string bean came up as weak for my system. Next, he put the chocolate in my hand and told me to think of joy and gratitude; the chocolate tested strong. So, the final thing I have to say on food is to eat with good spirit. If we eat with fear or strong emotions, the food will harm us. Consciousness matters.

While eating smartly leads to positive outcomes, rigidity and religiosity can be limiting to our health. The gist is to be free and in-

=themoment, to eat with connectivity. The trick to eating awareness is paying attention to how you are filling your tank, so that we have ample enough fuel to live well and enjoy what we eat. This is about developing common sense and critical reason.

Tools for health

Nature

Humans used to be forced into the elements in order to survive. It was taxing, but we were strong and hearty. We didn't have machines and computers. My grandfather had hands the size of baseball mitts and spent a lot of time working the land. He was tough as nails. Whether we exercise, walk, dance, play sports, or take a martial art, it is important to keep moving for our muscles and tendons (liver system), our blood circulation (heart system), digestion (spleen system), our immune system (lungs) and our bones and brain (kidney system). As you can see, we need to approach health as a whole organism. Another way for us to heal is to commune with nature. As we are of nature, communing with nature is a reminder of our cycle of life. Looking at trees, standing at the shoreline of a beach or lake can revive us. As we do with food, take in the colors, letting the elements of nature and their vibration feed your body, mind, and spirit. Personally, I find hiking restorative and centering. It incorporates the elements and minerals which nurture our bodies, a tremendous activity boosting one's metabolism, washing the senses with trees, rocks, streaming water, and the sun.

The Japanese call this Shinrin-Yoku or Forest Bathing. They did a study to assess the benefits of being in nature. "The findings were as follows. In the forest area compared to the city area, 1) blood pressure and pulse rate were significantly lower, and 2) the power of the HF (High Frequency) component of the HRV (Heart Rate Variability) tended to be higher, and LF (Lower enterocep Frequency)/(LF+HF) tended to be lower. Also, 3) salivary cortisol concentration was significantly lower in the forest area. These physiological responses suggest that sympathetic nervous activity was suppressed and parasympathetic nervous activity was enhanced in the forest area, and that "Shinrin-yoku" reduced stress levels. In the subjective evaluation, 4) "comfortable," "calm," and "refreshed" feelings were significantly higher in the forest area. The present study has, by conducting physiological investigations with subjective evaluations as supporting evidence, demonstrated the relaxing and stress-relieving effects of "Shinrin-yoku" (Tsunetsugu). Similarly, children allowed to play in nature have less anxiety, good study habits, higher grades, better health, and fewer psychological and developmental behaviors, says a study by Louise Chawla from University of Colorado. This applies even to urban kids who are exposed to parks or community gardens. When children are outside in nature, putting their hands in soil and climbing trees promotes an enhanced sense of connectivity and a willingness to protect the earth.

> Opportunities for children to connect with nature are important for the preservation of the biosphere. A large and steadily growing body of research shows that access to nature benefits young people in multiple areas of their lives. Reviews of thi literature show that when children have nature around their homes, schools and neighborhoods, it promotes their physical and mental health and cognitive performance (Chawla, 2015; Kuo, 2019; McCormick, 2017; Norwood et al., 2019; Tillman et al., 2018; Vanaken, 2018).

Nothing will make us understand the cycle of nature more than composting and gardening. We take soil and leaves from the ground in autumn, add ash from the fireplace to the soil in winter, and consistently enlarge the compost with scraps of organic food including corn husks and egg shells. Once the big, fat worms do their thing, the compost has the most wonderful earthy smell, rich in minerals, which provides fertilizer for our vegetable and herb garden in spring. We are utilizing the energy of all four seasons to begin the cycle of birth and growth again. I love the connectivity to the elements and seasons.

Another tool of health is to do things that let us receive light, or enlightenment. For example, learning something new or doing something out of our comfort zone can go a long way to a rich life. I recently taught a class that was live-streamed around the world. It was so out of my realm, but a beginner's mind enables us to grow towards mastery as long as we stay pure and wondering, never stagnant or static. I love being a student. I also welcome challenges which raise my frequencies. The self-expression of our authentic self through our pursuits leads us to a fulfilled heart. Knowing the laws of nature is often about common sense. As the ancients say, as we are nature itself, we already have the wisdom within us. It is my hope that you approach your everyday life, as purely and organically as possible, to be the healthiest, clearest, most vibrant you can be.

I am saying this at a time in our history when things are very challenging. We have been stuck in a pandemic, our lives on hold. As grueling as it is in present day, I always say it is one thing to thrive when times are good, but the question now is how do we find health and well-being when times are hard. More than ever, we need to double down on the principles of health, wellness, and spiritual fortitude. I think this time of global pandemic has given us great clarity to prioritize the things where we derive value in our precious lives and to discard the rest. It also solidifies feelings of gratitude for the things that bring us satisfaction. One way to honor ourselves is to practice self-care.

Self treatment (do-in)

Here are some tools to implement into your daily routine for optimal health. Dress comfortably,

A. You can sit on the floor in seiza (kneeling), cross-legged, or on a chair. Rapidly rub your hands together until it creates friction and becomes warm. Place your hands on your heart. Do this three times. Start with some upward motions with your hands on your forehead, beginning at the 3rd eye until you feel the area tingling. Put your hands on each eyebrow and press as you move towards your temples. Finish by pressing lightly on your temples. Do this three times (more if you feel tight).

B. Rapidly rub your hands together as you did before. This time, press lightly onto your closed eyes and leave the fingers there until you see light. Do that three times. You can do the same thing with your ears. Put your forefinger in front of your ears and the rest behind. Do an up and down motion.

C. Pay special attention to loosen the jaw. Open your mouth slightly. Put your fingers along your cheekbone, gently press, and move toward the outside of your face. You can stop and hold wherever there is tension. Put your hands on either side of your nose, moving them up and down. Press along your jaw line, above and below. Hold where there is tension until it releases. Put one hand above your mouth, another below, and move laterally in opposite directions. Press your fingers on your chin. Hold if there is tension.

D. Do upward motions on your neck. Do circular motions on your left shoulder, up and down motions with your upper arm, circular motions on your elbow, up and down motions on your forearm, circular motions on your wrists.

E. Press on the base of each finger and use the pressure to pull your fingers, much like cracking your knuckles (but without trying to crack your knuckles). Massage the inside and outside of your hand. Do the same thing on your right side. Open and close your hands on your chest. On your abdomen, if you are born female, move your hands to the left and massage in a circular fashion. Men go in the opposite direction, to the right.

F. For a kidney rub, put your hands under the back ribs and open and close to awaken the kidneys. Do the same thing on your pelvis.

G. Do up and down motions on the front and back of your thighs, circular motions on your knees, up and down motions on you calves and shins, circular motions on your ankles, up and down motions on your feet as you did with your fingers; pull the toes one by one all the way to the tip. Put your foot on your leg, massage the bottom of your foot with both hands like kneading dough, continue to press on an area that is sensitive.

H. To finish, go to your head and tap all over, including the back of your neck, the base of your spine. You can tap your face, anywhere. Put your hands together at the end in gratitude.

I have treated everything from structural injuries to chronic and severe illness. I see the effects of poor diet, stressed out lifestyles, long work hours, and dietary and alcohol excess, anxiety, obsessive thinking, and depression on the system. Meditation goes a long way to reverse the imbalance by bringing the mind and emotions back into balance. We address lifestyle, behaviors, diet, and all the influences that contribute to ill health and step by step as we go on the path to wellness. But, like any process, there are slips built in. This is not meant to be a rigid, punishing pursuit. We can find grace in the process of change.

Balancing emotions

Nakazono always said that the source of our anger and upset arises when we want something that we are not necessarily meant to have in that moment in time. As the poet Rumi says, "When I run after the thing I want, my days are a furnace of stress and anxiety; if I sit down in my own place of patience, what I need flows to me and with not any pain. From this what I understand is that what I want also wants me, is looking for me and attracting me. There is a great secret in this for anyone who can grasp it" (Rumi). A daily practice in mindful meditation allows us to experience spaciousness with the added bonus of living beyond or transcending the limits of our emotions. It also helps us release all the unnecessary phenomena which tether us to the world of illusion. Whether you do sounds, sit quietly, do hara exercises, or any of the many modalities and visualizations we can draw from, we will feel more aligned with the universe. If we can remember to turn our switch on to mindfulness as much as we can throughout the day, then we will heal. Of course, there is an ugly side to this. Spiritual practices can sometimes bring out our ego, feeling smug and superior: "Look at me, being enlightened!" Only nothingness in the here/now can abate our ego's tendencies. Let's not take ourselves so seriously. Laugh it off! We are not bound by dogma.

Perhaps music transforms us! Singing on the top of our lungs, dancing, crafts, art, a brisk walk with a friend, aikido, yoga, watching baseball, going to a concert, our path is our own to evolve and enrich.

When I lived in San Antonio De Las Minas, Mexico, I used to take my bokken and jo (wooden sword and staff) up a mountain with the local dogs from nearby ranches to do sword cuts and jo katas (forms).

This became my cleansing ritual. I love climbing up mountains just to feel the power of nature and to sit in solitude, at one with the flow of life. Purification rituals are endemic to many cultures. Baptisms come to mind. The Kabbalists write about the importance of Mikvehs, ritual baths for the purpose of purification. In Shinto, people perform Misogi, a purification which involves standing under a waterfall in a state of mindfulness. I once heard a story that Nakazono went to teach an aikido seminar in Montreal and did snow misogi, where he and his students stripped down and rolled in the snow as a form of spiritual cleansing. He used to suggest that at the end of a normal shower, make the shower cold and stand under it. Not only is it purifying, but it also invigorates and strengthens the immune system while improving circulation.

Clearing the body

Here is another self-treatment which also feeds your body, mind, and spirit. You can do this standing, seated, in seiza (kneeling), sitting cross-legged, seated in a straight-back chair or even lying down. This is the treatment I do on myself every morning, the way for me to put myself in the right consciousness, balancing my body and releasing the illusions I get myself caught up in before the day even starts. Take it as a clearing.

If you are standing, have your feet shoulder width apart, knees slightly bent, so that your back is in alignment. Tongue at the roof of your mouth. Eyes can be opened or closed. If you are in a seated chair, don't lean back. Keep your spine straight, yet supple. The pathway of energy within your body is like a spiral that is going up and down at the same time with every breath. The energy converges in the center point of your body, the hara or tanden in Japanese, approximately 3 inches below the navel. Take your mind and put it in your hara. Your

262

consciousness is now the center of our body. If you'd like, you can put your hands three inches below your bellybutton by cupping them against it. Breathe in through your nose very slowly, as slow as you can. You can feel your abdomen expand into your hands. When you reach the peak if your inhalation, hold, and then slowly exhale through your nose. Feel each microsecond pass within the breath. At the very end of the exhalation, hold, in order to empty your lungs and begin to inhale again. Clearing your mind, be in the nothingness. Once you feel ready, breathe into your hara and feel the energy or ki radiating out and up through your body. Let the ki permeate your body and cells. Your breath emanating from your hara is oxygenating your entire body. Pay attention to areas that hurt or feel tight. Breathe into the tight spots. Breathe into your bones, your muscles, tendons and tissue. Breathe into your eyes, ears, mouth, tongue, jaw. Breathe into your skin and feel the breath expanding out beyond your body, like a cylinder of ki. Then breathe, guiding your breath through your legs and feet towards the center of the earth. Form live roots out the bottom of your fee. Breathe as far as the center of the sky out of the top of your head. You can start with a few minutes a day, gradually increasing the time, so that you will do this throughout your day.

My aikido Sensei, Yamada Shihan always says as a matter of fact that you can be Zen anywhere, at any time, even or especially on a crowded subway train. I love practicing mindfulness on the subway, on the city street, everywhere at any time. Meditation is a way to drop into yourself, to go deep within. What can we do as humans to live a rich, fulfilling life? What can we do to live our time on this planet in optimum health? If we live according to the assumption that we are nature itself, we can rely on the elements of the universe to guide us to be our authentic selves. What does that look like? We have a physical form.

We have five senses, which are the antennae that perceive the world around us. We have our mind, which is the control center, the headquarters as it were. Lastly, we have our spirit, the purpose which drives our existence. Without soul, we are merely robots. If we prescribe that we are of nature, it would also stand that we are all part of a whole. The idea that we are divided or separate from one another is an illusion that over time has come to feel real. Our egos, in particular, like to differentiate our needs from those of other people. Our egos like to compete and compare. We judge. We want. We want more. A healthy ego has a sense of self, whereas a weak ego needs validation and separates you from me. It doesn't concern itself with the collective. It likes to be fed because it is hungry. The ego can be a great motivator, often the loudest voice in the proverbial room. And it often can drown out the soft breeze that is our soul.

Feelings and thoughts are mutable and in no way define us. Only we as the overseers of our own existence can put ourselves in balance by being the conductor of our own orchestra. How do we do that? We can start by moving through our feelings rather than negating them or sweeping them under the rug, only to have them rear their heads in the form of unconscious behaviors. It's beneficial to ask questions to make ourselves accountable. The Heart system is about awareness. Knowing our humanity, we ask, "to what extent are we enslaved by our story or the events of our past?" How does our past limit our growth? Can we let go of what we can't control? How can we use, even embrace these feelings as tools to our existence, but not let them damage our systems? Can we infuse a sense of radical acceptance to all that is, so that we stay in the flow of life? These conscious actions are part of the process on the road to balance. Excess emotion harms the liver and threatens our equilibrium. Each emotion can either be a catalyst for change or can be destructive. For example, fear has its usefulness. We learn to be afraid of putting our hands in fire, lest we burn ourselves. Sadness can awaken us to an unhealthy relationship, like a warning system, so we can take appropriate action. However, what happens to us when we let fear or sadness run amok in our system? We get anxiety and depression.

Clearing the day and preparing for sleep

To a practitioner of Eastern Medicine, sleep is also an important way to restore life energy and optimize the body's healing power. Ideally, if you can be fast asleep before midnight, earlier in winter, getting 6-8 hours of uninterrupted sleep gives you the best chance to revive. Unfortunately, insomnia and sleep irregularities have been a common complaint in my practice these days. Overactive brain activity from technology, worry, stress, alcohol, the news, rich food, sugar, all impair the quality of sleep. To improve sleep involves a multi-pronged approach.

For example, a study by Oxford University did a study that determined that insomnia is often caused by worries and anxieties that arise at night while we are at rest. They discovered that one is more likely to fall asleep and stay asleep if we write in a journal before bed to clear the mind and promote inner peace.

Patients with insomnia commonly complain that they are unable to get to sleep because of unwanted thoughts and worries. One account given of this excess cognitive activity is that it results from the incomplete processing of daytime stressors and hassles. Previous research has demonstrated the benefits of writing about emotional experiences as a method to facilitate emotional processing. This pilot study tested the hypothesis that writing about worries and concerns, with an emphasis on the expression and processing of emotion, will reduce sleep onset latency among an analogue sample of poor sleepers (Harvey, 1).

Scientists at Baylor University and Emory University of Medicine performed a sleep study that determined, more specifically, that a person who wrote a to-do list rather than a recap of the completed tasks fell asleep faster and easier. Additionally, making an effort to not ingest any food and drink (especially alcohol) after 8 pm helps the body prepare for sleep.

Prompts for journaling:

1. I am grateful for...
2. I forgive....
3. I'm feeling...
4. To-do list...

One way to clear the effects of the day is to sit, quiet your mind of thoughts, and be in your mind at your hara, conscious center, three inches below your navel. Give your mind a space vacation from overthinking and just feel life. You can follow your breath going from the center of the earth in the inhalation up to infinity and exhale from infinity to the center of the earth. Let the energy awash you completely. Slow down time to the microsecond. Release your thoughts and feelings. Let your spirit come home to its vessel. Just be. This is good to do in the evening or before bed.

Treatment starts with diagnosis, reading pulses on the wrist, asking questions. I palpate the abdomen, looking at the tongue, listening to the patient and the tone of their voice. For example, do they have a lung voice? This is the start of a profound process, as no two people heal alike. We are all the same and yet so unique at the same time; healing chronic illness or injuries therefore can be revealing and illuminating. Oftentimes, a patient has firmly established patterns of imbalance and there is a certain familiarity the patient might have with their illness or injury over time. It's the devil you know! Once we start to restore the body back to balance, we enter into a path together, guiding the body back to health, giving the system new messaging. Inevitably, there can be various points along the way where the patient feels stuck, often even more symptomatic again after a period of relief— discouraged, oddly protective, if not defensive of their sickness. This is often the phase in treatment when they start to doubt themselves, the process, and me. It reminds me of the moment during labor before the birth of the child, when the mother just can't go on anymore. She is experiencing the most pain at this time, the contractions at their strongest. This is usually when the cervix is in the process of dilating from 8 to 10 centimeters, referred to as the period of transition, the stage before the contractions change and the mother feels compelled to push. The transitional period is just this, the difficult moments before transformation. The same thing happens in the healing process.

I recently went through this with a patient who had eczema over his entire body. I recognized that he was suffering from an autoimmune response brought on by stress, anxiety, and diet. Needless to say, his skin appeared dry with a fiery redness and scabs from scratching himself silly. There came a moment after his treatments when he would feel relief, but his condition would revert back after a few days. This went on for some time. In the meantime, I muscle-tested him and concluded that he needed to eliminate dairy, which was difficult due to the fact that he was vegetarian, and not vegan, and struggled to get enough protein intake. I also prescribed a mixture of Chinese and Western herbs to his regiment. At one point, he said to me snappily that those herbs were not helping. I got it!! It sucks!! I told him to be patient and persist. He would need to be on them long-term. I could tell he was getting frustrated. It was right around the time of COVID, before everything stopped. He was feeling sick, and his skin worsened. He took baths in the middle of the night, in agony from itching. It was further drying his skin. He had a persistent cough, chest congestion. His throat hurt. His jaw was tight. He was not a happy camper. Then, one day, I read his pulses as usual and noticed that his condition had changed. For the first time in months, I needed to address a different system. The chain was unraveling. At the same time, his skin was looking good. He was healing.

When Sensei Nakazono started treating me, my pulses and my symptoms indicated an imbalance of my heart/small intestine system. In addition to abdominal pain, I had circulation issues, cold hands and feet, muscle stiffness, and my intestines were inflamed. After a few months of treatment, dietary changes, probiotics and other herbs and supplements, meditation, sound practice, and inner work to forgive and clear the past, I got really sick. I had fever. I had pain all over. I couldn't leave my bed. After a couple of days, I was back to myself. When I went for treatment, my diagnosis changed. The healing crisis was the culmination of my commitment to biopsychosocial wellness. I felt better than I had since I was a little girl. I was evolving on the road to healing.

Healing requires work inside and out. Everyone is different. However, to live pain free, to bring your body into balance, to change a pattern of behavior, to heal, requires fortitude, patience, resilience, and self-love. Pain, in and of itself, is a guide, a teacher which sends us on a process to find the balance we seek. These days, in my practice, I see a lot of patients with varying degrees of anxiety, from crippling and self-sabotaging to a general malaise. It has become commonplace.

When we are in the flow of the universe, our consciousness offers us a balanced way to experience the same phenomena. Feelings limit us, plus they are steeped in illusion. I can feel one way about something

268

My Eastern Paths to Healing

and, with some space, feel the opposite way a day later. Critical thinking, which I call the overseer, is the mindfulness to see what is real. Letting the overseer, the totality of us in the moment, question our limited beliefs systems, emotions, and patterns, can go a long way towards truth. This is what this book is about, to put us on the side of life, to make us whole. To unify our parts is to overcome their pathology to do us harm.

Joy and Compassion

To develop our emotional intelligence means to understand the fluidness and fleetingness of feelings, They don't create our identity nor even what's real. But they can be self-induced. For example, the emotion related to the heart system is joy, something we can generate from within. We need not wait for the world to make us happy. I mean, yeah, Kettle potato chips make me pretty darned happy, albeit temporarily. Because internal joy, like the warmth of summer, is expansive, putting ourself in that frame of mind attracts light from everywhere. One exercise that I recommend to access joy is to think of something or someone that makes you smile. Put the smile in your heart and the center point in the middle of your chest, between your breasts. It is the energy center of your spirit, your shen (Chinese) or shin (Japanese). Breathe into the point and back in the smile until it fills your body. Another way to attract light in our life is through compassion and sharing.

In Eastern medicine, the cycle of human life is such that from conception to birth, children are connected to their parents' life energy, specifically their mother's. Females are on a 6-year cycle and males are on a 7-year cycle. When a child enters into my practice, if the girl is 6 or the boy is 7, there is a chance that I would have to treat the mother as well. When a girl turns 12, or a boy turns 14, their energy converts

269

from one of receiving into one of sharing as contributing members of their community. Their life energy is expanding out as they begin to relate to and interact with the world around them. By the time kids reach adolescence, they are oftentimes more invested in interactions with their peer group, forming their lifelong identity. Sharing is medicine for our heart, the language of love.

If you were to meditate on the word "compassion," how does it feel in your body? Where do you feel it? Can you feel it in your heart area? A nice guided mediation you can do to strengthen your spirit is to breathe into the "shin" point and heart. Feel the center of your chest open like the sun shining in the noon sky. Next, feel the same sun shining from the point in your back. Then, have the sun radiate down towards the body and up through your head. How can you share? Can you conduct yourself with grace? Can you inject space into a situation before you blow up? Can you breathe?

Are we enlightened yet? Healing ourselves changes the life energy of the universe. Nakazono Sensei talked about that often. As we subsist off the land, made up of the same elements, if we truly know in our cells that the earth is us, would we be less inclined to threaten it? Would we protect her? We can start by being present and practicing self-care. It is up to us to create our reality, to be in the silence where our true selves can emerge, our soul integrating inside our bodies as its rightful owner. What I experienced back in 1985, when I dropped everything I'd thought made me who I was and instead immersed myself in this "new" path of life, as old as life itself, still fuels me to this day: the mind-bodyspirit connection, that we are nature, the essence of creation, the infinite that is and our finite expression of it. Most of life to its source is both mysterious and unknowable. It even eludes the poets, the scientists, and the philosophers. Yet, the Ancients preserved wisdom for us which tells us we have the intelligent capacity to heal ourselves. As the universe seeks balance, so do we. Pain tells us when we veer off course, giving us the opportunity for change. I can never properly express my gratitude for being on my ongoing path to biopsychosocial wellness and the drive to guide others to do the same. In the midst of this are the place keepers of the ancient ways, the information for a transcendent life path. Just the coming together of this book, with the fusion of different perspectives of a single imperative towards holistic health, shows the push forward to a new paradigm, a way of unifying healing, interconnected, as one. Perhaps this is just the collective we need to tackle life's ills while making life meaningful and transcendent. Journey on!

WORKS CITED

Chawla, Louise, "Benefits of Nature Contact for Children." Journal of Planning Literature, 7/22/2015
https://doi.org/10.1177/0885412215595441

Harvey, Allison G. and Clare Farrell, "The Efficacy of a Pennebaker-Like Writing Intervention for Poor Sleepers." Behavioral Sleep Medicine, 1:2, 7 June 2010, 115-124,

Kuo, Ming, Michael Barnes and Catherine Jordan, "Do Experiences with Nature Promote Learning? Converging Evidence of a Cause-and-Effect Relationship." Frontiers in Psychology, 19 February, 2019.

McCormick, Rachel, "Does Access to Green Space Impact the Mental Welleing of Children: A Systematic Review." National Library of Medicine, Sep 4, 2017.

Nakazono, Masahilo M., The Source of Present Civilization, Kototama Books. Dec. 1994.

Ni, Maoshing. The Yellow Emperor's Classic of Medicine: A New Translation of the Neijing Suwen with Commentary. 1995

Norwood, Michael et al., "A Narrative and Systematic Review of the Behavioural, Cognitive and Emotional Effects of Passive Nature Exposure on Young People: Evidence for Prescribing Change." University of Bath, 2019

Rumi. Rumi Poetry: 100 Bedtime Verses. Createspace Independent Publishing Platform, 2017.

Scullin, Michael K. et al., "The effects of bedtime writing on difficulty falling asleep: A polysomnographic study comparing to-do lists and completed activity lists." Journal of Experimental Psychology: General, Vol 147(1), Jan 2018, 139- 146.

Tillman, Suzanne et al., "Mental Health Benefits of Interactions with Nature in Children and Teenagers: A Systematic Review." Journal of Epidemiology and Community Health, Vol 72, Issue 10, 2018.
Tsunetsugu Yuko, et al., "Physiological Effects of Shinrin-yoku (Taking in the Atmosphere of the Forest) in an Old-Growth Broadleaf Forest in Yamagata Prefecture, Japan." Journal of Physiological Anthropology, Vol 26 (2007) Issue 2: 135-42.

Vanaken, Gert-Jan and Marina Danckaerts, "Impact of Green Space Exposure on Children's and Adolescents' Mental Health: A Systematic Review." International Journal of Environmental Research and Public Health, Vol 15, Issue 12, 27 November, 2018.

van Leer, Bernard, The Beginning of Life (Documentary).

***** For a comprehensive list of Five Element Theory, Sound practice, or Do-In videos, please visit **www.kototamalifetherapy.com**

CHAPTER XI

Yoga: Empowering Your Health Through Your Inner Evolution

Dr. Marisa Galisteo

Welcome to my Chapter! I am honored and grateful that you are here!

Since I was a little girl it's been my deepest desire to support and empower people's physical health and their overall well-being. So much so that I declared as a 9 year-old that I'd some day make a pill that would cure cancer and thus would help millions of people worldwide to be happier. However, in my own winding evolutionary journey I've come to the humble realization that the source and power to healing and to sustainable health and well-being does not lie outside the body but rather, it exists within.

My intention for you is that this Chapter will effectively support you in bringing forth a new, radical relationship with your health and well-being, and one that you can sustain for the rest of your life. How I am going to support you in achieving that is through a twofold model:

1. Enlightenment: Specific coaching distinctions that help you reveal your inner truth.

2. Embodiment: Specific practices with breath work at their core to help you embody your revelations and to directly support and empower your innate wholeness.

Enlightenment:	Coaching distinctions
Embodiment:	Energy Codes Breath work practices and BodyAwake Yoga

This is what transformation is: a revelation of truth—in an 'A-Ha' moment— that naturally brings the release of illusionary beliefs that have kept at bay the abundance, the wholeness, and well-being that we truly are and have. Rest assured that wherever you are in your own healing and empowerment journey is absolutely perfect. In whatever ways you are ready, open, and willing to listen to and integrate the teachings I bring you here, you will. As such, I am starting this Chapter sharing key aspects of my own personal journey, with the intention that they bring light to you and your own unique journey.

Section 1: My Own Personal Journey

Ever since I was a child, my heart saddened as I saw people suffer, and it's been my heart's desire to become someone who can effectively help millions of people to be happy. I've also been forever fascinated about how life works: Isn't it amazing that planet Earth gives us everything we need to live and thrive? Isn't it amazing that we can move around without being plugged into an outlet? How do the ~30 trillion cells in our bodies work, both individually and together to keep the entire body functioning properly?

So it may not be a surprise to you that at the age of 9 I declared to myself –and to my dad—that I'd find a cure for cancer. Achieving this goal would allow me to relieve suffering for millions of people on Earth, and restore them to their well- being and happiness. At that time I believed it would take a lot of effort, but it was definitively possible. And my dad believed it too! He would encourage me on Sunday mornings at   the kitchen table—where I'd sit right after waking up to study science— telling me that I'd get the Nobel Prize some day. Seeing him be so convinced that I could accomplish that was so empowering to me!

I spent my days and nights studying and learning, walking my path towards college. A strong knowledge of chemistry would be necessary to develop a successful drug against cancer, so I went on to major in Chemistry. Being involved in research led me naturally to do a Ph.D. I joined an internationally recognized research group at the University of Granada (Spain), where after 4 years I obtained a Ph.D. on Biophysical Chemistry of Proteins. A couple of months later at 26 years-old I became a professor there and started teaching one semester a year to senior students. I loved teaching my students! During the rest of the year I performed research on folding and assembly of viral capsids as a Visiting Scientist at the Department of Biology at MIT (Cambridge, MA). This would end up being my 'bridge project' between my Ph.D. and finally doing research on cancer specifically.

I was accepted to work at a highly competitive laboratory at NYU Medical Center, with Prof Joseph Schlessinger, one of the most successful scientists in the field. They were already making great progress on the elucidation of some of the molecular and cellular mechanisms that are deregulated in cancer. Joining this lab was a dream come true, even though it meant leaving my position as a professor back in Spain. At NYU I spent 7 years learning and using the most highly specialized molecular biology techniques. The work required many skills, from the intellectual understanding of my projects to the fine work with my hands. I loved working in the lab, designing experiments and doing all they required. Very good at this highly creative and intellectually stimulating activity, I published 7 articles in peer reviewed journals during that time and have published a total of 15 in my scientific career. It brings me great joy to see that some of my publications continue to be cited to this day, 20 years later.

My boss moved his lab to Yale University in July 2001. One side of me was thrilled that now I'd be able to spend much more time with my daughter, who was 18 months old at the time. However, I was also heartbroken, having fully dedicated the previous four years to a highly sophisticated project that did not produce the kind of striking results that would have granted its publication in the kournals Cell, Nature, or Science. And it was quite clear that my chances of ever going back to the lab were slim.

I fell into a depression with an identity crisis, not knowing who I was. I did not realize at the time that I was suffering because I had attached 'being a scientist' to my identity and that if I had known that, and had released that attachment, I would have given myself freedom. This is a perfect example of what healing and empowerment can look like and what this Chapter is about!

My son was born 10 months later. As I continued to unconsciously expect happiness to be delivered to me from the outside, my marriage started to tremble. During that time of my life I hid from the world: did not tell my family, and did not reach out to any of the few friends I had; I was too embarrassed of who I was and about what my world was, self-perceptions that I did not want anyone to know. I felt completely alone with my misery, and hired a therapist just to have someone to talk to. She put me on anti-depressants, which deepened my feeling of being a loser, all of which I kept as a secret from my family and the few friends I had. During this very painful period of my life I did not know that a different, empowered, joyful and creative life was possible. At least not for me. I was being a complete victim of my circumstances, which, as I now know, corresponds to the lower part of the spectrum of consciousness that I've depicted in Figure 1.

In early 2004 I had a key realization (enlightenment!) that took me out of the void I had been in for almost 3 years: "Intellectual stimulation is what I've been missing!" This led me to NYU Career Services and to start taking classes on management and all kinds of topics (including 'English Writing' with Bob Davis!) at NYU SCPS (School for Continuing and Professional Studies). What struck a chord big time for me was my class on Foundations of Coaching. I learned there that coaching is about helping others fulfill their potential, to facilitate the positive change that is required to achieve goals that are truly worth going for. Sitting in that class and hearing coaching's purpose caused me to experience a powerful 'A-Ha' moment: Being someone who gives people access to fulfill their potential felt completely true for me! I could not believe my ears! My heart was finally singing after 3 years of dark silence, and I was thrilled to start training to be a coach!

A few months later and as my divorce process began, I came across Yoga. I really did not know anything about Yoga, other than it could possibly help me with stress and posture, but felt I needed to experience it. Little did I know then the degree to which it was going to change my life! So there I was at my first Yoga class: going to the back of the studio to hide, I sat on the mat crosslegged as everyone else but I started to feel very uncomfortable right away, and I looked in the studio mirror and saw that my back was rounded, when everyone else's was straight. I didn't know what was going on, but plenty of self- criticisms such as "I am different," "I am broken," and "I don't belong" voiced themselves all at once. The class started and I was having great difficulty following instructions; I couldn't breathe and barely could do any of the poses.

Half-way through the session I found myself hyperventilating, and had to stop. It seemed as if yoga was 'impossible' to do. However, somewhere in my being I sensed that there's "medicine" here for me. I immediately hired a private Yoga teacher and started working with him right away. The first thing he taught me is how to breathe. How come I did not know how to breathe?!

I started to have countless 'A-Ha' moments both on the Yoga mat and off the Yoga mat because of my regular practice on the mat. Looking self-love, and compassion. At the time, I did not have the distinctions of Enlightenment and Embodiment, but now I know that that is what I was experiencing then: I was slowly but surely discovering more and more of my inner truth, and my life started to become more aligned with my truth.

Practicing Yoga and deepening my coaching studies became priorities for me, and in the next few months I established a collaboration with David Rock, one of my Coaching teachers at NYU SCPS, and I began to do research on the relationship between how the brain/mind works and coaching. This exciting research was used in the book Quiet Leadership that David was writing.

By the time my divorce process was complete, I had clearly experienced in my being that Yoga practice is a powerful practice not only to help with posture and flexibility, but for raising consciousness and for catalyzing personal transformation and becoming a more loving human being, so I naturally wanted to share it with others. I registered for a Vinyasa Yoga teachers' training program at my local studio, at the same time that I was learning NLP (Neuro Linguistic Programming) to further my coach training.

I came across Kundalini Yoga just a few days after I graduated as a Vinyasa Yoga teacher, fell in love with it, and also registered to do the

Kundalini Aquarian Teacher's Training. During this time I also was traveling to attend Yoga retreats with world-renowned teacher Shiva Rea and others, and also meditation retreats in the US and France with Thich Nhat Hanh. What a privilege to get to learn directly from these Masters of Consciousness!

I started teaching to small groups of friends in my home in 2008. I also started teaching at Yoga studios but found it not as fulfilling; I discovered that it's important to me to personally connect with my students and follow their personal evolution. Teaching Yoga and coaching came together in a beautiful way as an integrated effective path that was healing and empowering me, as well as my students and clients.

In 2010 I participated in a transformational coaching program that allowed me to experience multiple 'A-Ha' moments and shifts in consciousness that allowed me to access and release illusionary beliefs, resulting in extensive forgiveness of self and others and access to more self-confidence and self- love than ever before, all in just three days. And just as with everything I find powerfully transformational in my own experience, and inside of my calling to give people access to their own empowerment, I immediately started to train to lead the program. This training typically takes several years, and with the intention to speed up the process in 2016 I took on a job as a full-time staff member, which I felt as an honor and a privilege. This job was the perfect training ground to learn and develop effective management and leadership practices as well as to cultivate my ability to making an even larger difference in people's lives. And little did I know that taking on this job was going to catalyze a major spiritual awakening!

Eighteen months into this position I started to develop a frozen shoulder. As months passed the pain intensified and the mobility of my left shoulder decreased so much that I had to stop doing my favorite physical exercises: Yoga and swimming.

Getting dressed in the morning was an excruciating experience. For many months I did not connect this pain with being in the job. Gradually it started to became a hint that grew louder and louder. At some point it became quite clear that this pain was a message telling me that remaining in this job was no longer aligned with my truth and that it was time for me to leave. However, I kept convincing myself that I needed to stay, with the main reasons being 'not wanting to look defeated,', fear of losing the appreciation of a like-minded community, and not wanting to disappoint the many people that were counting on me to stay in the job. Now, looking back, I can see that all of my reasons had to do with fear of being judged and, specifically, fear of losing others' love and appreciation. It's a very natural human reaction that is sourced by the ego or protective personality fighting fiercely for its survival.

The longer I went against my truth by staying in this position, the more my suffering intensified and the harder it became to do the job. Now looking back, it makes total sense! As I now know, the Soulful Self tirelessly waits for the mind to catch up, and sooner or later the light of its truth will shine on and melt the workings of the ego/false self. So, I finally surrendered and resigned, and the surrendering itself was the transformational action that took me into the Void.

Three months later the Universe presented me with the work of Dr.Sue Morter; her first book, The Energy Codes, had just been published. I started listening to the audible version and, as I listened to her words, I was moved to tears with one A-ha after another! My heart felt so 'at home'! Dr. Sue, as she likes to be called, is all about empowering people to master their health and their lives, from the inside out,

281

through embodiment practices. She has developed the Energy Codes (EC) principles and practices to give us effective access to a radical and sustainable transformation. This transformation is accomplished by activating dormant circuits in our electromagnetic energy and nervous systems (more on this later). Said in another way, this transformation is accomplished through embodiment practices that integrate mind, body, and breath together.

This powerful quantum technology was my new path in front of me, and I felt so joyful and grateful! Not only that, a couple of weeks later I found out that she'd developed her own Yoga style that integrates the EC practices into Yoga: BodyAwake Yoga. I went "OMG" and immediately registered for the Teachers' Training. And then, after over a year without being able to do any Yoga because of the pain and lack of mobility in my shoulder, I gathered enough courage to go on my Yoga mat and attempt to come into downward facing dog. My pose was highly asymmetrical due to my shoulder's condition, and tears of sadness and joy were running down my forehead. I continued to practice a little bit every day, incorporating the specific breath work from the EC while on the pose. That together with gentle swimming and receiving a specialized form of physical therapy helped me heal faster, regaining mobility and strength in my left arm again. By the time the BodyAwake Yoga Teacher's Training Program started in Oct '19, I had only about 5% left to have my shoulder back to normal.

In March '20 the Covid-19 pandemic hit and I realized I had with me a technology that could tremendously help the people who were in their homes frightened and not exercising. I found myself 'jumping in the pool,' nudged by my soul, and started reaching out to people and live- streaming four Yoga classes a week. Since then to this day I've livestreamed over 200 BodyAwake Yoga classes to students in 11 countries. The summer of 2020 I 'threw myself into the pool' again, when I started teaching BodyAwake Yoga in Spanish. The idea of teaching Yoga in Spanish had crossed my mind in the past,; however, every time I dismissed it, mainly out of fear that I might freeze often during teaching, whenever I would not know how to translate a word or guide my students throughout the class effectively. I've now taught over 60 classes in Spanish. In this last year I've also become a certified Facilitator and a certified Coach of the Energy Codes, and I've been working with individuals and groups in those capacities in English as well as in Spanish. What a joy and what an honor to contribute to the lives of these amazing human beings!

I invite you now to take a moment and be in this inquiry: What aspects of your life's journey are you finding that are mirrored by my journey? Can you see that moments of suffering in your life have also been catalysts for spiritual awakening and expansion and have supported you in finding what's next for you?

I have great news for you! There is no need to suffer anymore to catalyze this process! Embodiment practices that help us cultivate our innate wholeness are the answer. This will be covered in detail later in the Chapter. First, let's explore how we can connect with our inner truth:

Section 2: Coaching distinctions that help you reveal what's true for you: Enlightenment

As I shared in my own journey above, we human beings have developed a protective personality or ego since childhood, giving rise to a false self that wants to please others to avoid judgment and to be loved. The limiting beliefs of unworthiness that define the false self are stored in our body, our energy field, and our subconscious mind. Our life's choices are driven by these protective patterns at least 95% of the time, and "Until you make the unconscious conscious," as Carl G. Jung noted appropriately, "it will direct your life and will call it fate." For you to live a more consciously created, freer and happier life, you will want to unveil what's really true for you, behind the mask of the protective personality. As this updated version of reality emerges in your awareness, your choices will be more congruent with what's true for you.

An effective way to shed light on what's really true for you is using coaching distinctions, linguistic constructs that allow for revelations of your inner truth as 'A- Ha' moments of insight. In effect, they help us bring what's subconscious ('from the dark') to conscious awareness ('to the light'). We all have experienced those moments: it's as if a light bulb went off inside your head! Therefore, coaching distinctions support the raising of your consciousness by inducing clarity, revealing to your awareness a new piece of what's true for you.

Different transformational programs offer their own specific coaching distinctions, even though many of them are basically the same, just named differently. In this section I've gathered some of my favorite coaching distinctions that are very effective in helping you reveal more of what's true for you. There are also coaching questions intermingled in the text. Thus I recommend that you have your lap top or a notebook and pen nearby, so that you can capture your revelations. I really hope you find it highly user-friendly and get back to it often!

In this section and in the chapter overall I'll use interchangeably Soulful Self, Higher Self, and True Self to refer to our divine aspects vs. our human aspects.

The first distinction that I want to bring to you is:

1. VICTIM vs CREATOR

We are VICTIMS when we believe we can't do anything about the situation we are in (powerless). At the other end of the spectrum of consciousness, we can be CREATORS and create our own experience and outcome independent of the external world (empowered). A bit more conscious version of victim is when we are hopeful that our life can get better; we may seek therapy or self-help courses during this stage. It's the beginning of your awakening!

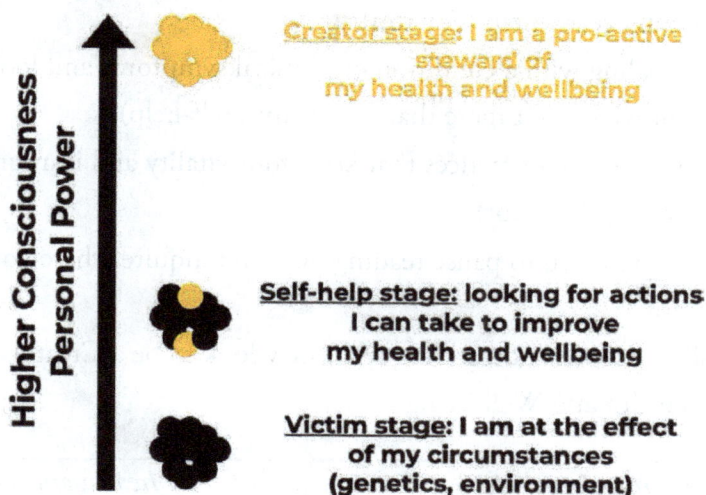

Creator stage: I am a pro-active steward of my health and wellbeing

Higher Consciousness
Personal Power

Self-help stage: looking for actions I can take to improve my health and wellbeing

Victim stage: I am at the effect of my circumstances (genetics, environment)

I invite you to take a look in your own life: you probably can identify some specific areas or situations you are dealing with right now where you're currently feeling like a victim (e.g., being inside of the Covid-19 pandemic at the time of my writing this chapter), and other situations/ areas of life where you are trying to fix something and maybe resolve something with others when you are being the creator of your life experience.

Notice, in your own experience, that as you move from victim to creator in more and more areas of your life, you're elevating your consciousness and experiencing more and more moments of freedom, selflove, peace, and joy, together with a life where there's more flow. When it comes to the area of your Health and Well-being, where are you at in that scale?

Here are some examples to help you look:

- Dealing maybe with a chronic condition that does not heal and being hopeless about it, continuing to take drugs that don't really help? (Victim)
- Dealing with a condition or physical symptoms and looking for what's out there that may help? (Self-help)
- Doing daily practices that keep your vitality and immunity strong? (Creator)
- I invite you to pause reading now and inquire where you are at.

A possible statement describing what may look to be a Creator in the area of Health and Well-being is:

> *"I am responsible for (and the creator of) my health and well-being. I am responsible for creating the environment inside of myself and around me that will support my staying healthy throughout my life."*

That may sound like a big leap for most people at this time. And that is what I am interested in bringing to you: A radical empowering of your wholeness.

This leads us to the next distinction:

2. CONTEXT = your "come from"

I define Context here as a belief or set of beliefs that give you a particular lens or filter to look from and look through whatever is at the forefront of your awareness. The contexts we operate inside of are mostly subconscious. They originated at very early ages when we faced moments of 'failure' and decided things such as "I am not good enough," "I'll never be X, Y, or Z," etc. These limiting beliefs create a false version of who we are. They shape and color what's actually happening in front of you, and automatically generate a particular meaning in your awareness which comes with particular feelings in the body, and will lead to specific actions/choices resulting in a particular outcome. So, every outcome in your life is correlated to and comes from a particular Context. I also invite you to notice when you look at your own experience how there was a complete absence of love and trust in the moments in which limiting beliefs were generated.

Take a moment to look for yourself. Limiting beliefs are therefore coming from the reality of the FALSE SELF. This distorted view of reality takes the shape of wrong assumptions about ourselves, others, land ife, and often will lead to a great deal of suffering for ourselves and others. These false beliefs affect the electromagnetic energy field of the body, distorting its flow and causing energy to get stuck in the body. And the energy associated to the feelings that we don't embrace is pocketed away in the body's tissues (defense physiology). Energy stuck in the body will sooner or later produce physical symptoms and ultimately disease of the body (Morter, 136).

Here are a few common examples of limiting beliefs and the impact of believing them:

1. While you believe that you don't deserve to be loved, you won't perceive love when people around you are loving you and you'll likely feel lonely and suffer.

2. While you believe you are not capable of becoming the leader that you know you are, you'll experience yourself as small and you'll suffer.

3. While you have a dream that you don't believe is possible for you, you won't manifest it and you'll suffer.

Maybe after reading these examples there's a limiting belief of yours that has brrm revealed to your awareness?

If of course you are operating from beliefs that are TRUE (natural laws, universal laws, cosmic laws), then your context is going to be one that empowers you, and the correlated actions will produce miraculous results in your life.

Here are a few examples:

1. I am a sovereign Creator of my life.

2. Everything that happens in my life is in support of my highest good.

3. My life's purpose is to bring more love to the Planet.

You may want to take the opportunity at this moment to bring to your awareness something that's currently challenging in your life, and I invite you to look at it through any of these 3 lenses. You'll gain a new perspective on it that empowers you and you'll find yourself taking new creative actions towards solving it. As you can see, different contexts result in very different life experiences. That is why it's key to examine both the context and the beliefs that are running your life, making them conscious. This is what the process of 'awakening' is. The statement I wrote above, coming from being a Creator, "I am responsible for (and the creator of) my health and wellbeing. I am responsible for creating the environment inside of myself and around me that will support my staying healthy throughout my life," is a consciously created 'come from' or context that provides a new way of relating to one's health and well-being. If I choose to believe that statement because it empowers me, my actions will be correlated with it. So, if someone offers me a can of soda, the action that's aligned with this consciously created context is for me to say, "No, thank you." And I won't have to think about it. No effort. My reply will arise within me organically. That is the power of context. Therefore, the context, the 'come from,' what we believe, determines our choices, including our choices regarding our health and well-being. If we don't create our contexts consciously, they'll be created for us by our subconscious, which is filled with limiting beliefs from past experiences and other people's beliefs that we unconsciously took on as 'ours.'

What's your current context for your health and well-being? Have you created it consciously? Most of us have not. We did not even know about context! We may not even know that my choices regarding my health and well-being may be coming from what I learned watching movies and TV shows!

How you find out about your context in the area of health and well-being is by looking at your daily choices of food, drink, air your breathe, exercise, sleep, and thoughts. I invite you to pause here and start to make a list. Then brainstorm some possible contexts that empower you (feel free to use any of the three I offered you above) so that you consciously choose/create your own choices. Always create contexts as statements/declarations in the present tense, and make sure that you feel empowered by them. And if my statement above resonates strongly with you, feel free to make it your own!

When you are ready, move on to Distinction #3:

4. EXTERNAL vs INTERNAL OR INNER ORIENTA- TION

"Where attention goes, energy flows. Where intention goes, energy flows." -James Redfield

External: We human beings don't realize how much we are externally oriented. It may be obvious that we are using our 5 senses to receive information from the outside world; after all, that's what they are for. However, having an externally oriented focus has us look outside of ourselves for the things/people we believe we need in order to experience the freedom, love, joy, and peace we all seek (as I shared in My Own Journey section above).

How much time in the day DO you spend with your attention focused on your cell phone? And your lap top? TV? There's an App that counts how many hours and minutes a day you are on your screen, if you are curious to accurately know. But for now, just estimate. How many hours? Besides the hours, what are you watching? What are you feeding your conscious and subconscious minds with? What 'juice' are you getting out of this overloading of your senses? Notice if you already are feeling 'wrong' about it. There is nothing wrong. But by taking inventory of the reality of what you are doing, you get to observe your patterns and therefore to elevate your consciousness. This new, updated reality—which is much closer to reality than your previous perception— may lead you to take a new action or even a new habit (see Chapter III) that supports your health and well-being.

This external orientation also supports a victim disposition, since if the outside world does not deliver what we want, we feel bad, sad, anxious, depressed. And as our energy is projected outward, by the end of the day we are so exhausted and wonder why. Inside of this external focus we also tend to notice and point out what's not working, what is wrong or missing that needs fixing. If all we do is live life with this external orientation, what are we not experiencing? Foremost, the wholeness that we are! The vitality and joy that our cells are made to radiate! And this vitality and joy is precisely what we've been seeking, looking for in all the wrong places, outside of ourselves!

Internal: The importance of re-directing the mind's attention to the inner world is already described in ancient yogic texts and termed Pratyahara. Pratyahara is usually translated as

"withdrawal of the senses" and more literally means "gaining mastery over external influences," which frees the mind to attend to the inner world. Swami Sivananda tells us that "Pratyahara itself is termed as yoga, as it is the most important limb in yoga sadhana."

There are a number of simple practices which we can do to practice Pratyahara and which create positive impressions in the mind:

- Turn off your electronics or put them in silence mode and close your eyes and focus on feeling your breath.

- Go out in nature and practice gazing at the horizon, a forest, a lake, an ocean, the blue sky... or practice being present with trees, rocks, flowers, etc.
- Visit temples, use altars, candles, incense, etc. to alert your mind that it's time to go inward.
- Yoga, and particularly BodyAwake Yoga (see below). Another key distinction that's related to this External vs Internal orientation is:

LIVING IN THE HEAD VS LIVING IN THE BODY

When you wake up in the morning, where are 'you'? You likely experience yourself somewhere in or around your head, don't you? I mean, you don't wake up and find yourself inhabiting your knee, or your hand, or your foot. You are in your head and that's where you live.

Therefore, we make feeding our mind with knowledge and information a priority. And of course we feed the body when we are hungry, but other than that we largely ignore the body. And ignoring the body results in a diminution of life force or Prana, twhich will eventually cause symptoms and even diseases.

Even if you are exercising the body you may not be doing it consciously, as when watching a TV show while running on the treadmill. Nothing wrong with that— however, you are not in the body and therefore are unable to enjoy all the benefits you could get for your health if you were to bring consciousness to walking or running on the treadmill. What does it look like, then, to be in the body, you may wonder?

"Being in the body" is directing your mind's attention to the body, to any specific areas/tissues where any sensations are felt, no matter how subtle, and recognizing that what you are feeling is the energy that you are. This is a beautiful mind-body partnership that when coupled with conscious breathing through the area where you are experiencing the sensations, results in integration of mind-body-breath, which is the formula that allows for experiencing the wholeness that we are; this, therefore, is what needs to become our priority. The integration of mind-body-breath is also one of the definitions of Yoga, and it is what you will accomplish through the Energy Codes embodiment practices: a new health and wellness paradigm that focuses on cultivating the wholeness that we are. Regarding 'being in the body,' there is an invisible and magical part of you, your central channel: a column of energy running across your body from the top of your head to the tip of your spine, also called Sushumna in Sanskrit. This central channel is home for the 7 chakra system, the place in your body where your life force resides in its highest concentration. Isn't this something that you really wanted to know about but didn't even know anything about? We want to master tapping into this infinite source of wholeness, which will result in healings in all areas of our life. That is what we do with the Energy Codes embodiment practices, directing our attention inward to the central channel and cultivating its presence. This brings us to Distinction #4, whose subtle differentiation helps us better understand the invisible power of the Sushumna:

3. INVISIBLE ANATOMY VS PHYSICAL ANATOMY

This segment will act as a bridge between the Enlightenment and Embodiment sections.

It is a belief for most of humanity that who we are is the body (physical anatomy) that has a mind and a soul, because it is what we can see with our eyes. And therefore all will be over when breathing stops. In other words, we identify ourselves as the body/mind. However, besides our obvious physical anatomy, there is a subtle—and very exciting—realm not visible to the eye: the etheric body, the chakra system. There are 7 chakras within the body, from the tip of the spine (chakra 1/root chakra) to the crown (chakra 7/crown chakra). They are vortexes of energy or energy centers in the body, each of them corresponding to a different level of consciousness. These are the chakras that are familiar to most people, but I'll mention in passing that we also have less-known chakras—8, 9, 10, 11, and 12—outside of the body, corresponding to even higher levels of consciousness and vibrational frequency. We activate, balance, and integrate all of these chakras (1-12) when we practice BodyAwake Yoga, which I'll expand upon later in the chapter.

The chakras are also connected with the ~72,000 nadis (Johari, 2010) and the meridians —super-fine pathways through which energy travels within the body. The chakras may be invisible to us, but when they are partially or totally blocked, this imbalance has a profound impact on the body: sooner or later we'll experience pain, inflammation, and even diseases in the body.

I personally have known about chakras since I began my first Yoga Teachers' Training back in 2007, and have visited them in many trainings since then, but I never knew how to make that knowledge useful in my own life in any way, shape, or form. Through my studies with Dr. Sue Morter and the Morter Institute for BioEnergetics I now know how to work with the chakras to support my health and well-being and I am sharing it here with you. In the following Table I've gathered information about the chakras that's relevant for our discussion.

CHAKRA	Symptoms	Consciousness	Breathwork and other practices	Yoga poses
1st (Root) chakra, base of the spine	Mental lethargy and spaciness, osteoarthritis, poor general health	"This is my life, and I get to choose my experience moment by moment." "I belong." Vibrant health	Mula Bandha Central Channel Breathing	Chair pose, Warrior I, Pyramid pose, Tree pose, Standing forward fold
(Sacral) chakra, just below the navel	Feelings of isolation, impotence, low back pain, prostate and bladder issues	"I create joyful relationships and my communication flows with ease." Development of intuition.	Take it to the Body	Boat Pose, Pigeon Pose, Yogic Bicycle, Seated Spinal Twist, Breath of Fire
3rd (Solar Plexus) chakra, base of the sternum	Digestive issues, stomach ulcers, allergies, diabetes, chronic fatigue	"I allow my own way and I allow yours." Confidence, self-esteem, power.	B.E.S.T. Morter March	Camel Pose, Bow Pose, Reverse Table Top, Crescent Warrior, Breath of Fire
4th (Heart) chakra, center of the chest	Codependency, shallow breathing, high blood pressure, heart disease, cancer	Love and compassion, vulnerability "Everything is in my favor." Abundance.	Heart Coherence Breath Generating Loving Presence exercise	Triangle Pose, Thread the Needle, Fish Pose, Reclined Spinal Twist
5th (Throat) chakra, base of the neck	Perfectionsim, inability to express emotions, sore throat, thyroid issues, neck aches, asthma	"I hear and speak the truth with grace and ease."	"I manifest easily." Breath patterns for Healing	Cobra Pose, Plow Pose, Bridge Pose, Toning with Sound (Om, Ma, Ha)

| 6th (Third Eye) chakra, middle of the brain | Nightmares, glaucoma, headaches, learning difficulties | High intuition. Perceives beyond the 5 senses, creative genius | Saliva pH to gauge alkalinity in the body Conscious Exercise and BodyAwake Yoga | Downward Dog, Shoulder Stand, Child's Pose, Peaceful (Exalted) Warrior, Balancing Poses |
| 7th (Crown) chakra, to of head | Depression, confusion, epilepsy, Alzheimers' disease | "I am a divine being." | Central Channel Breath Meditation | Corpse Pose, Headstand, Rabbit Pose, Wide Angle Forward Fold |

*Information for this table has been mostly extracted and curated from Morter, 76-77.

In the first column we find the name of each chakra and location in the body. The text has been highlighted with the corresponding chakra color. In the "Symptoms" column we find common symptoms and types of illnesses. In the "Consciousness" column there are some examples of statements that we'd say when the corresponding chakra is operating at its highest power. In the "Breath work and Practices" column I've listed one breath work and one other practice for each chakra. There are more practices in The Energy Codes book for each chakra. I've selected two per chakra here to keep it simple. In the "Yoga Poses" column we find some poses that focus on the activation of the corresponding chakra.

HOW TO USE THIS TABLE TO SUPPORT YOUR HEALTH AND WELL-BEING:

For example, if you have a heart condition, you'll find that it is a symptom of the heart chakra not functioning properly.

So, you'd go to the "Breath work and other Practices" column corresponding to the heart chakra and find that the recommended practice is the Heart Coherence Breath and the Generating Loving Presence exercise. In addition, it's important to realize that the heart condition is a symptom and the cause of the symptom may reside in a different chakra. So you will also want to ask your body: "Is there any other chakra related to this symptom that I need to work on?" Sense and feel your body for the answer and go to work there!

Section 3: Embodiment Practices that Activate your Innate Ability to Heal And Empower your Wholeness

When we have an 'A-Ha' moment, we are in the presence of so much clarity that we believe we are never going to forget it. But I bet you've had the same 'A-Ha' more than once. Why? The light that was present in the first moment of insight was not embodied; it remained at the level of the mind, only. In order for transformation to be sustainable, we must embody our revelations. What follows is a selection of specific practices for embodiment, which help integrate mind, body, and breath together as one. They allow for empowerment at all levels of your being, beyond your physical health. I've made a selection of some of the embodiment practices described in The Energy Codes book, focusing on 1-2 practices per corresponding chakra (as in the Table above). It's been challenging to choose, since each practice is so meaningful and empowering. For more detailed information on these practices and for learning about all the others that Dr. Sue has developed, go to Dr. Sue's book The Energy Codes. Rather than starting with Chakra 1 and going one by one to Chakra 7, I'm going to place my analytical mind to the side, allowing my true self to present this information 'out of order' and to start with Chakra 4, heart chakra. Why? Because your loving presence resting in and moving through your body is the healer within: "To heal the body, we have to be in the body. To heal most powerfully and quickly, we have to be in the body in love" (Morter, 185). It's important that we are in the vibration of love and joy while we do the practices.

At some point, with enough practice, being in this vibration of love will be your 'come from' rather than your 'go to.'

Chakra 4:

Love is the healer within. For most of us, the love that we are used to experiencing is conditional. This is a natural result of wanting to protect our heart from getting hurt. Loving this way is also an experience of attachment: when I love you, and you love me, you must stay. It's as if you belong to me. However, "When we land in the core of our being, love is easy to experience because it's what we're made of " (Morter, 186). Further, and in fact, "The magnetic field produced by the heart is more than 100 times greater in strength than the field generated by the brain and can be detected up to 3 feet away from the body, in all directions" **(HeartMath Institute). (To access fascinating research on the heart-brain- emotions connection, visit: https://www.heartmath.org)**

Generating Loving Presence Exercise (Self-Love):

Things or people external to us can and do activate the vibration of love within us. This is why we tend to think that the love we feel is coming from them, when the truth is that their presence happens to activate and reveal the vibration of love within ourselves. This exercise will give you the experience that the love you feel is generated by you and received by you and, therefore, unconditional. This is how to do it:

1. Start breathing in your belly, and allow high frequency energy from the cosmos to pour through

    2. your crown down the center of your body. Allow yourself to receive   this energy, cosmic intelligence. You realize you can choose how to use this energy.

    3. Now think of something that you love. Something that brings love and joy every time you think of it. Perhaps it's your beloved and the gratitude that you feel for having this kind of connection in your life. Or it could be your pet, or your best friend. Or the magnificent view of a sunrise or a sunset over the ocean. Feel this love and appreciation. Imagine you are eye-to-eye with this. Let yourself be loved back as you are loving it.

    4. Notice how you feel in the body and turn up the volume of these sensations: keep loving it, let yourself be loved back, and notice how it melts you in the inside. Continue to amplify this feeling, letting it emanate off of you, even bigger than the room you are in. Notice how it feels in your body, and memorize it.

    5. Now place your hand on your heart and claim it all for you. Whisper to yourself, "this is for me"; all of this energy is rushing in and you are now receiving it. Feel it. It's unconditional love, since you've generated it and you're receiving it. Feel this love that you have generated.

This is the love that now you know is possible. This is your self-loving presence. You can memorize it and return to this vibrational state as often as possible. Practice all the time, even while doing the dishes or driving down the road. Allow it to be your 'go to' until it becomes your 'come from.'

Heart Coherence Breath: The breath of the Cosmos

This breathing pattern has become one of my favorites to practice daily. I also love to bring it to my BodyAwake Yoga classes, particularly when we are holding downward facing dog. This is how to do it:

1. Visualize a sphere of golden light all around you (at least 4 feet radius).

2. Begin to inhale, drawing the high frequency light from the sphere, from all directions, into your belly (in front, behind, right and left, above and below).

3. As it enters your belly, start to move it up the central channel, passing through and stretching the solar plexus, and opening the heart. Keep inhaling as the light (it's you) continues to be drawn upward towards the upper lobes of the lungs. Keep inhaling even bigger than the body. Now exhale long in all directions.

4. Repeat as many times as you want. I do at least 3 cycles. This is, by the way, the most simple and effective breath to relieve anxiety and stress.

Chakra 1

This is our anchoring chakra. Its activation helps us come down from the head into the body and anchor on the Earth. It helps us feel safe, complete, and at home, as we integrate mind, body, and spirit.

Mula Bandha or Root Lock:

The activation of Mula Bandha is similar to Kegel exercises, requiring a contraction of the muscles of the pelvic floor. It's a lifting up of the pelvic floor muscles towards the navel, as if we're drawing energy from the Earth up into the body through this section of our body. At first, if you are new to this, you may need to contract all the muscles in the pelvis. It's totally OK. Practice makes perfect. Try it now and notice how you feel in the body. With this practice we easily anchor our consciousness into a single point and we feel grounded and stable instantly. We are awakening those tissues with life force and establishing a new—higher—vibration in that area of the body. This will become a simple, instantaneous practice that will change your life! Practice as often as you can during the day! There are 3 additional anchor points, at the heart, throat, and third eye chakra levels. Engaging the 4 anchor points at once is a key practice of the EC that effectively helps us embody our consciousness.

Central Channel Breath (CCB):

This is the foundational breath of the Energy Codes. Imagine a funnel that opens up to the cosmos on the top of your head and becomes a channel through the center of your body, to the tip of the spine. Now, get yourself seated in your heart, activating the vibration of love within you, maybe visualizing an image of a person or something that brings you lots of joy. As you are feeling that way, now inhale as you let high frequency light (your Higher Self) pour down through this funnel and enter through the top of your head down the center of your brain, center of your throat, center of the chest, to your belly; let your belly expand with this breath, then begin to exhale drawing the navel to the spine down the tip of the spine and into the Earth.

Now start the breath from within the Earth, inhaling to the belly, letting it fill with high frequency light (Soulful Self) and exhale rising up through the channel and out the top of the head. As you consciously follow the breath, inch by inch, you are activating all the circuits along the path. This is a whole cycle of CCB. Repeat as many times as you want.

In summary: you breathe in from beyond the body to the belly, and exhale out to beyond the body, in one direction first, then the other. As you do this breath, you are activating the presence of your Higher Self in your body, rejuvenating yourself and drawing cosmic intelligence onto you. As you become more and more familiar with this breath, you'll find yourself doing it anytime anywhere. You'll no longer 'kill' time: any open time can be used to give yourself the gift of the benefits of practicing CCB.

Chakra 2

This is our wisdom center and also our feeling body. This feeling body refers to the physical feelings, or sensations we experience in the body, which correspond to movements of energy. When we label our sensations as good or bad, pleasant or unpleasant, we are in duality and being conditional about them: We like the good ones and we don't like the bad ones. However, they are all energies. So, this resistance or rejection to feeling certain energies that arise in our body is what causes the short-circuits in our energy field that will likely end up leading to physical symptoms and disease. Only when we get to embrace ALL OUR ENERGIES will we be able to heal and experience the wholeness of our being.

It's paramount that we learn to work with ALL THE ENERGIES that arise in our system, particularly those that we have labeled as 'bad.' Dr. Sue discovered that the sensations that arise in our body when we are experiencing a charge, like a knot in the stomach, or tightness in the chest, are pointing us to where in the body we have a short-circuit, a gap in the energy flow. It's our Higher Self talking to the mind through the body. Knowing this allows us to work with these energies in a very effective fashion towards healing our system. We accomplish this with the practice of "Take it to the body," which is why I consider this practice foundational to the Energy Codes and foundational to anybody's health and wellbeing! This is how to do it:

Take It To the Body (TITTB):

Whenever you feel emotionally triggered by a person or circumstance, rather than going to your head, come into the body: There will be a place in the body where you'll feel a charge.

First, note:

1. where in the body the sensation is,
2. what the sensation feels like (hot, cold, pressure, buzzing...) and
3. what chakra may be the one affected.

Then,

1. go there with your consciousness and love, and
2. squeeze the area from the inside, as if you were hugging it, intimately, as if taking care of a frightened child.
3. Then begin to breathe up and down the central channel with as much love as you can generate, integrating this area into the channel flow until you feel a shift in the energy. It will probably take at least 4 complete cycles of CCB.

For those of us who have been living in our heads all our life, it maybe hard to feel where the charge is, simply because we have not been living in that area of the body and the circuits responsible for letting us feel that area are asleep. If that's the case, you can ask your mind (with as much love as you can), "Where do I need to activate circuits in my body so that I can be with this situation without getting triggered?" Whatever the first place where your mind lands, trust that that is the place.

I suggest that you start to get familiar with this practice when you are calm, and consciously with your imagination bring in front of you a person or situation that typically triggers you in some way. Practicing in the 'in between moments' is how it will eventually come naturally to you when the challenging moment shows up. And fewer challenging moments will show up!

This practice can also be used to work towards healing any painful area that already exists in the body. Consider that the area is painful because, as a result of a gap in the circuitry, the stuck energy is over-stimulating the surrounding tissues, which may be causing inflammation and/ or may have already manifested as a chronic condition. So, give this painful area a loving squeeze from the inside, tell it that you are 'moving back in' as you breathe up and down the channel, activating the circuitry for health and wholeness in the area. And don't forget to ask: "where else can I build circuits in my body to relieve this pain?"

Chakra 3

When something happens that is really upsetting to us and we reject it, resist it, and are unable to embrace it, a short-circuit is created in the energy field, and the energy flow stops there. And then that area of the body starts to show a disfunction: "What starts as an energy issue eventually becomes a tissue issue" (Morter, 158). To manifest a vibrant life, we need to start to accept life as it comes. You may say, "I may be able to do that moving forward, even though it does sound challenging enough!" "And … what about all of the short-circuits that already exist in my energy field from all the times I've resisted life? What can I do about those?" To answer the latter question, that is precisely what all the Energy Codes practices do: All of them reconnect this disconnected circuity. This is the path towards self- healing and self-empowerment.

B.E.S.T.: BioEnergetic Synchronization Technique

In this section I want to bring your awareness to the existence of this healing technique, developed by Dr. Sue's father in the '70s. A pioneer in energy medicine, he developed B.E.S.T., which is a very powerful hands-on, self-healing technique. During a B.E.S.T. session, a number of circuits that were short-circuited due to the rejection of stressful events get reconnected again, and the moment the energy starts to flow again as designed in the body, self-healing occurs. "We are rarely stuck always something deeper that is really the cause" (Morter, 159). I also want to mention that there is a self-administered version of B.E.S.T. called B.E.S.T. release. It was developed jointly by Dr. Sue and her father and you can find it in Morter, 168-174.

Morter March:

The Morter March is a powerful practice that helps us heal from traumas. It activates and unifies multiple areas in the brain and systems of the body at the same time, thereby creating a reset of the nervous system that allows us to release emotional unresolvedness from our subconscious and to replace it by a new message to the subconscious with the sense of well-being and love that we want to feel. This is how to do it:

1. Stand with your feet hip-width apart and your spine straight and tall.

2. Step forward with your right leg, bending it into a lunge, with the knee over the ankle. Back leg remains straight.

3. Place both hands together in front of you and lift up your arms to about a 45-degree angle. Now, lower your right arm until it's back and behind you at a ~45 degree angle, pointing to where the wall meets the floor. Notice that your right thumb is pointing down. Extend all the fingers awake.

4. Tilt your head slightly to the left shoulder and look directly up to your left thumb. Close your right eye.

5. Standing in this position, allow yourself to feel a deep sense of wellbeing, and then take a deep belly breath and hold it for as long as you can. Then exhale and step back with your right leg.

6. Repeat on the left side. And then once more on each side. This life-changing healing practice is recommended twice a day, first thing after getting out of bed and last thing before going to sleep, since those are the times in the day when the communication between the subconscious and the conscious mind is most enhanced.

Chakra 5:

The throat chakra governs our breathing, our ability to manifest, to speak our truth, and to listen to others. We are going to bring mind, body, and breath together, as we place our attention in a particular area of the body and we breathe through it. This is how we activate self-healing.

There are specific breath works that allow for activation of each of the chakras (see Chapter 8 of the Energy Codes), but in this section I will focus on teaching this one powerful healing practice called:

Breath Patterns for Healing:

> "Pain exists in the body because of a lack of energy flow
> through the affected area" (Morter, 226).

With this powerful and elegant breath work we'll be able to start to move energy through any area requiring restoration of proper energy flow and the integrity of that area. Let me give you a quick overview of the practice first, to make it easier: With the affected area squeezed, you'll inhale from beyond the area to the heart, being the light that's moving through the body, as if 'stripping the area through with healing light,' followed by an exhale out the other end of the central channel.

This is how to do it:

1. To begin, let yourself get into the vibration of your loving presence, as best you can.
2. Now, choose the area you are going to work on. Come inside that area with your consciousness, with your loving presence, with intimacy, tenderness, and care, as if hugging a frightened child.
3. The first inhale is from beyond the area to the heart. Squeeze the muscles along the route and stretch them at the same time. This may take some practicing, it's all good! For example, if it's your left shoulder, extend your arm out to a position where you can feel enough intensity, then inhale through

307

your fingertips, up the arm (being inside the tissues and as if you're the energy that's being drawn with the breath—you actually are) through the painful shoulder, to the heart, then exhale down the central channel and into the Earth.

4. Next, inhale from within the Earth to the heart, and exhale through the painful shoulder (continue to squeeze and stretch the muscles along the route) down the arm and out the fingertips.

5. Now, you could take a regular central channel breath as described under 'chakra 1.'

6. Repeat steps 3, 4, 5 several times as needed.

This breath work can be used for any part of the body that hurts or does not feel totally healthy.

Thousands of people have had remarkable healings doing this practice. And you can, too!

Chakra 6:

The third eye chakra is associated with the pineal and pituitary glands, which are in the center of the brain precisely where the cerebro-spinal fluid is made and from where the chemistry of the body is managed. I'll now summarize a couple of very important practices that contribute to a healthy third eye chakra:

Nutrition and Saliva pH:

The cells in the body need an alkaline environment to thrive. When the pH is too acidic, they begin to die. "Ninety-five percent of all diseases occur when the body is in an acid state. Cancers are the extreme result of a highly acidic state" (Morter, 238). So, we want to keep the body in an alkaline state, which is the state needed for healing and rejuvenation. No wonder the 40 years of research on nutrition that Dr. M.T.

Morter Jr. did showed that, to facilitate healing when inflammation or disease is present in the body, our diet needs to contain ~75% of fruits and vegetables. Measuring our saliva pH regularly allows us to monitor the alkaline or acidic state of our body in a very simple and quick way. Additional recommendations are presented in Morter 244-250.

Conscious Exercise and BodyAwake Yoga:

As I mentioned earlier in the chapter, most people while exercising are either watching TV on the treadmill, or listening to music. Nothing wrong with that, but those activities distract our mind from focusing on the body. Dr. Sue has trained professional athletes and champions to break their own records by the simple practice of doing CCB (as described under Chakra 1) while they work out. As you do CCB, you're drawing high frequency light into your core, therefore tapping into a larger quantity and quality of energy than when not breathing this way. This allows you to do more in less time and without fatiguing. When Yoga is practiced with this conscious awareness in the central channel, we have the most robust combination of healing and wholeness practices all in one: That is BodyAwake Yoga. See below the last segment of the Chapter for a detailed description.

Chakra 7

Chakra 7 is about our connection with God Source, Spirit, or Higher Self. Energy medicine techniques work with moving the energy in the body. Something that's unique about the Energy Codes practices is that we identify ourselves with this energy that moves up and down and through the body. This energy is our true, essential self, and its presence in the body—its embodiment—is what we are cultivating with the energy codes practices. We want to learn to still the mind so that the true self can rise through the very noisy mind and we can perceive it with the mind. There are several practices that activate this chakra and help us still the mind. One is the CCB that I taught in 'Chakra 1.' Another is:

Meditation:

There are many kinds of meditation. I am going to focus on a type of meditation that's very easy and even fun to do, where you chant along a Sanskrit mantra. Chanting mantras may be easy and is incredibly powerful, because not only do these mantras still the mind, but they are also vehicles or pathways for commanding transformation, as we focus our dispersed consciousness into the sound waves of the Higher Self. There are many amazing artists who specialize in chanting mantras. My favorite ones to listen to and chant with are: Deva Primal & Miten Snatam Kaur

The two mantras that I feel the most joy chanting are:

1. The Gayatri Mantra

Mantra for enlightenment. Roger Gabriel tells us that "All of wisdom, knowledge, and the entire Vedas are concealed in the 24 seed syllables of the Gayatri Mantra." For detailed information about this mantra, go to: https://chopra.com/articles/the- gayatri-mantra-for enlightenment

2. OM Tare Tuttare Ture Swa-Ha

This is the Green Tara Mantra and has the power to liberate us from our attachment to suffering.

For an in-depth description and understanding of the power of this mantra, visit "The Sophia Code" by Kaia Ra, 132-138

BODYAWAKE YOGA/SUMMARY/CONCLUSION

In this chapter you have become aware of and learned of the importance of being in the body and of cultivating the integration of mind-bodyspirit to support your healing and sustain vitality and optimal health. You've become aware of and learned simple and powerful practices that can be done anywhere, anytime, and that allow you to activate the circuitry responsible for your healing and wholeness—a pioneer technology for self-healing and self-empowerment that does not require anything from the external world. The fact that most of these practices can be done seated, standing, or even lying down makes it even easier. That is pretty amazing! Whether you are already a yogi or not (yet), you don't want to miss the fact that when we move the body while doing the EC practices, we get to activate more circuits, faster. And if the movement involves putting the body in sacred geometries— Yoga asanas—even more so! Yoga asanas are specific shapes we can put our bodies in that allow our energy to rush through the body in specific ways and directions that support our wholeness. In BodyAwake Yoga we make this process conscious, using visualization to direct our awareness to the flow of energy up and down the central channel and consciously rushing high frequency light— unconditional love—to and through the specific areas in the body that feel tight, begging for love and healing. Pocketed emotions that were stored in the tissues as a result of traumatic experiences causing emotional and maybe even physical pain for many years can now be released, and energy can flow freely through that area, again resulting in healing right there on the mat. You are healing your inner child while on the mat! You are letting go of illusionary beliefs and re-writing your past while on the mat!

Consequently, with BodyAwake Yoga we not only become more flexible, stronger, and faster, but catalyze our own healing process exponentially. It is the most robust combination of healing and wholeness practices all in one. Because of all these benefits, practicing at least a few minutes of BodyAwake Yoga daily is my #1 recommendation towards cultivating your healing and well-being. If you are not a yogi, or if your body feels tight and your poses don't look like those in books, it's totally OK. You can still do BodyAwake Yoga. What matters is your desire to support and sustain your healing and vitality throughout your entire life.

~ ~ ~ ~ ~ ~ ~

To learn about my online and in-person coaching and Yoga offerings for individuals and groups as well as to explore co-creating a personalized wellness program for you or your organization, you can reach me at marisa@marisagalisteo.com

ACKNOWLEDGMENTS

I want to dedicate this Chapter to my parents: To my father, who recently transitioned (1932-2021), for his never-ending joy, for always believing in my potential, and for his loving support not only for me but for everyone who crossed his path during his time on Earth. Te quiero, papá. And to my mother, for her passion for learning that was passed down to me, for her dedication to her children, her love and support, and for being my mom. Te quiero, mamá. I want to express my heartfelt gratitude to each of the multitude of outstanding teachers and students that have come across my path so far and have contributed to my awakening, my healing and empowerment, and to my becoming a more loving—and happier—human being. A special gratitude note for Robert Davis for his continual support and encouragement all these years since we met at NYU back in 2005, and for trusting that I could be a qualified contributor to this book.

WORKS CITED

Gabriel, Roger, and Deepak Chopra, "The Gayatri Mantra for Enlightenment"
https://chopra.com/articles/the-gayatri-mantra-for-enlightenment

HeartMath Institute, "Science of the Heart: Exploring the Role of the Heart in Human Performance"
https://www.heartmath.org/research/science-of-theheart/ **energetic-communication/**

Johari, Harish, Chakras: Energy Centers of Transformation. Rochester, VT, Destiny Books, 2000

Morter, Dr. Sue, The Energy Codes: The 7-Step System to Awaken Your Spirit, Heal Your Body, and Live Your Best Life, Simon & Schuster, Atria Books, 2019

Ra, Kaia, The Sophia Code: A Living Transmission from The Sophia Dragon Tribe. Mount Shasta, CA: Kaia Ra & Ra-El Publishing, 2016

Rock, David, Quiet Leadership: Help People Think Better- Don't Tell Them What to Do: Six Steps to Transforming Performance at Work. New York, NY: Collins, 2006

CHAPTER XII

Practical Pilates for Every Body
Greg Grube

Pilates is a comprehensive exercise system with an extensive history. It has the potential to positively impact every area of the body that benefits from actualized and visualized physical movement. If you have never tried Pilates as such, chances are you have done some semblance of it or sampled some pieces borrowed from the vast array of exercises that harkens back to the 1930s. In that respect, it is time-tested and continued to be informed by the broad expansion and appreciation that physical exercise now has in contemporary life. What was once novel and experimental is now commonsense and backed up by research.

It is widely claimed that in Pilates there are more than 500 exercises and innumerable variations. Since every body is uniquely proportioned and idiosyncratically developed, the movements are tailored, often in real time, to those individual needs. One universal truth I hold as a teacher is that the better you seem to get at Pilates, the more challenging the work becomes on multiple levels. Going right to the edge of one's physical point of control is instrumental to building strength in Pilates. Muscles that start to shake and tremble, for example, indicate that the body has the potential to create a stronger neuromuscular connection to underutilized muscles that have already been developed. Imagine tapping into strength that usually remains dormant. Myogenic development, on the other hand—the generation of new muscle fibers—is durational, taking three months or longer. Pilates can help integrate these two important modes of strength building.

Another tenet is that basic movement fundamentals are present, utilized, and reinforced throughout the system. As these movement principles are drilled and attempted with varying degrees of success, a thoroughly embodied logic begins to permeate the practice: it becomes systematic. We know it is true that progressions and regressions complement each other to develop strength, stability, mobility, agility, balance, and all our other goals. Regression is the simplest form of a complex dynamic movement. If doing a push-up is difficult, then regress to just the plank position or place your knees on the floor; if walking is difficult, work on simply pointing and flexing through your feet. At root, Pilates helps us feel and look better as we advance though our lives. Like yoga, it is certainly a lifetime practice and can be successfully utilized at every stage of one's physical and psychological development.

Resting, Assessing, and Making Headway

One of the best ways to start a Pilates session is simple and effective: "Lie down on your back, knees bent, feet flat on your back, arms at your side." Then, a few specifics: heels lined up with the sitting bones, and the center of the knees lined up with the hip sockets. If you find satisfaction in this level of detail, that's good news: there's much more to come. Thankfully, our nervous systems respond to novel experiences and feedback, which helps us tune-in and make positive changes more readily. If you are already a seasoned practitioner, and this is familiar ground, then the intimacy you have attained can be comforting and you can infuse it with self-generated cues and imagery. Pulling in positive material from other practitioners with whom you've learned or from information you've read can yield powerful results. For example, you might couple the bio-mechanical imagery with information learned about how to break your negative neurolinguistic conditioning about a "frozen" shoulder or those damaging self-perceptions about your weight and age. Merging source material helps us create something unique to address the true idiosyncrasies of each individual.

The other benefit of starting simply is that pupils have an immediate sense that they have already done something well. We don't want to give empty praise, but positive reinforcement tends to have a greater impact than its opposite. By resting on the ground, we've already accomplished something impactful and have started reaping the benefits of dedicating time to this endeavor. The floor specifically provides ample support for the spine and the limbs. The back of the head and back of the pelvis are automatically aligned, which is something we can then aim to find when we're standing or sitting. Surplus weight and pressure are taken off the supporting structures between our joints, including our intervertebral discs. Overworked muscles have a chance to reset so that we can start finding support from muscles that might be underworking or are inhibited.

Before any intentional movement begins, the pupil and the teacher can fill this container, what is commonly called the Constructive Rest Positions (CRP), with a range of imagery, information, questions, and suggestions that can prime us to move better. Here's a partial list of nine of those cues to practice.

1. Visualize a very clear centerline: nose, sternum, navel, public bone, space between the knees and the ankles aligned. Couple the idea of the midline with the idea of a central axis, thevery middle of the body, our true cores. In other words, the body has a right side and left side. It also has a front and a back. It may sound obvious, but exploring the body in this way through movement can yield some profound results: anytime we veer off or away from center we are like a structure whose parts don't stack up. This means, ultimately, that we'll have to apply an

excessive amount of effort over time to maintain what's already less than optimal positionally, which can lead to overly contracted muscles, strain, and heightened tension—all things we want to lessen in the body.

2. Imagine the downward slope of the thighbones (femurs) pouring down and resting into the hip sockets. Visualize the hips as being deep sockets, and the head of the femur fitting and floating in the acetabulum, the socket of the hipbone. Refining our sense of the shape and size of our own joints can help us clarify our movements and untangle less helpful embodiments.

3. Feel the 26 bones in each foot spread into the floor. Do the same things with the hands —note the extra bone in the wrist—and remember that our fingertips and toes are dense with nerves, which is why they are so sensitive to touch. The hands and feet have varying degrees of dexterity, but in general there's a fair amount of brain space allocated to what happens in distal points. Later, initiating and reaching fully through our extremities can help us activate entire muscle-chains more fully: reaching away from our centers pulls us back together.

4. Widen the back of the pelvis and the sacrum, the triangular bone just below the lumbar vertebrae. Visualize the front of the pelvis narrowing— especially on the exhale. Finding a neutral pelvis can be thought of as a three-step process—pubic bone level with the floor and ceiling, hip bones parallel to one another, two sides of the pelvis evenly weighted like scales.

5. Commit to the inhalation. A five-count breath functions nicely with work that comes later. Try breathing into the abdomen and the chest simultaneously. Breathe front-to-back, side-to-side, and top to bottom. Sense how the air entering the body is

cooler than the air leaving the body. Notice the gentle stretch of skin and fascia as the body expands—how the spine elongates, how it calms the nervous system, how it lengthens the spine. For an added layer, visualize the heart beating slightly faster on the inhale and slowing down slightly on the exhale.

6. Find equal weight across the right and left side of the body. Check in with the back of the head, back of the rib cage, and back of the pelvis specifically. Balance the two sides like you would balance a set of scales.

7. Reach through the fingers' tips gently and press the palms of the hands into the ground to check in with the back of the arms and upper back. Widen across the collar bones and roll the shoulders gently back. Instead of pulling the shoulders down, allow the shoulders to elevate subtly on the inhale to allow more room for the lungs and ribcage to expand. Let the shoulders rest down and spread out on the exhale. There's no need to pull or jam your shoulders into position.

8. Proprioception is our awareness of where are bodies are in space—many of the cues above rely on fine tuning how the body is oriented in space. On the other hand, enteroception is an awareness of what's happening internally. The awareness of our heart's beating, or bringing our attention to the organs and glands including where they are located inside the body can be especially useful: the ascending colon on the right, the descending colon on the left. The liver underneath the lower ribs on the right, the spleen on the opposite side. Focusing on the internal organs can also precipitate a shift to a parasympathetic state, where we are able to rest, digest, regenerate. The body really is

a vast and remarkable universe that we should be learning about on an ongoing basis, not just when something goes awry.

9. In addition, orient your body in time and space very specifically. Notice the room you are in, its dimensions and features. Bring your focus to the mat or the equipment you are lying on. Know that we function and express ourselves in an environment, never in a vacuum. It's how we interact and connect with things that matters. This might be termed exteroception, how we interpolate external stimulation into our internal landscape. Combining all this sensory information gives us better stretch, helps us increase strength, move with more grace and fluidity. We want our whole being involved in the movement, giving ourselves permission to take up more space; to move like animals or elite athletes is part of this integrating process. Even though there are many times where we look piecemeal at the body, be certain to take some time to live, breathe, and feel the organic oneness and wholeness of your own body.

In addition to these generalized cues, the first five or ten minutes of a session can yield a vast amount of information, and additional cues can emerge on the spot to address the particular imbalances in the body.

Funny head tilts, scoliotic deviations of the spine, muscles gripping extraneously are some common dysfunctional patterns that can be addressed here. This is also an opportunity to converse freely. We certainly do not need to be stoic about our aches and pains.

We don't want to reify or reinforce pain structures through an internal or external dialog. Self-fulfilling prophecies notwithstanding, one of our main goals is to have the experience of something having been improved in a short period of time. By acknowledging and affirming that something's been ameliorated, that something just feels a little better, we can potentially work our way out of the labyrinth of chronic pain.

The Impetus to Move

The question of where to begin is always paramount. One unique feature of the Pilates method is that there are always multiple entry points. There are a number of what could be called closed-systems that intersect with more open-ended approaches to the work. These approaches, not mutually exclusive, ensure that we don't get bored or run out of challenges.

For example, the original mat work developed by Joseph Pilates himself is comprised of roughly 34 exercises that are completed consecutive to one another. His book Return to Life is still the definitive text for what truly constitutes Pilates as such, which was originally called Contrology.

The set sequences can easily be modified, exercises can be omitted as needed, and contemporary approaches have created a layered or tiered approach so that there are beginner, intermediate, and advanced levels within the larger scope. The same holds true on the piece of equipment known as the Universal Reformer or on the Cadillac.

Another truth is that Joseph Pilates was a consummate inventor. A fully-equipped Pilates studio has a vast array of equipment, props and tools, which indicates that even the progenitor of the method was aware that for many people a one-size fits all approach would not bring about the desired results of a uniformly developed body. The use of springs or straps to help people accomplish things that they are not able to on their own exemplifies this. Assistance, sometimes called spotting, helps make us stronger as much as actual resistance does.

Still, the best place to start is always with the basics, the fundamentals, which are a container that we can fill with the vast storehouse of human movement potential. Sometimes this is called pre-Pilates. Here listed are ten useful basic or fundamental exercises from the repertoire:

1. Position the head on the floor so that the crown of the head extends to the wall directly behind you, nodding the head gently to create a gentle stretch and release in the back of the neck. The heads sits on top of the spine somewhere between the ears and behind the nose, and we attempt to move the skull on the very first cervical vertebra. Above all, this should feel good. Turning the head slowly side-to-side and circling the nose on the ceiling can be very beneficial in restoring balance around the neck muscles.

2. Reaching the arms up to the ceiling, imagine the back of the shoulders resting onto the floor. Visualize the top of the arm (the humerus) as a little ball resting on the floor; some people call this plugging, but let gravity and the weight of the arms help make this more sustainable. Notice the movement potential in this position: little circles, turning the upper arm in and out, we can also try reaching the arms back overhead, taking the arms into a big T-shape, and reaching the shoulder blades around the sides of the ribcage to protract the scapula intentionally. All of these movements can become further refined as you make additional progress.

3. If spinal flexion hasn't been contraindicated as in osteoporosis or cervical herniations, then curling the head, shoulders, and chest off the mat is a cornerstone of the Pilates work. This does not mean that Pilates is out of the question for people who need to keep their heads down. However, if you can lift up, try taking the hands behind the head and peeling off the mat one bone at a time. If you come up for 2 counts, hold for 2 counts, and

lower down for a slow 4- counts, you'll tap into all three kinds of muscle strength—concentric, isometric, and eccentric. The upper back muscles release nicely when this movement is well executed, and it is a great way to start strengthening the abdominals.

4. From the head, let's move to the tail and think about the ways we can move the bones of the pelvis. Visualize the pelvis as a sphere and roll it back and forth, toward your chest and then to your toes. We call this action tilting the pelvis. Of course, the nomenclature (posterior and anterior tilt) is less important that feeling and sensing the movement. Common language like tuck and untuck works just as well as any technical terms for some people. I encourage people to do this exercise if as many ways as possible. Try it with some gluteal activation—squeeze the butt a bit, then try it another way, by curling the tailbone and lifting up through the pubic bone. Play with the feet pressing down, the heels pulling back. Come up a little higher and lift the pelvis and a few of the low-back (lumbar) vertebra off the mat. Improvising subtly within the form is often the best way to ignite new strength.

5. Picking the legs up is one of the first things infants do before they find the strength to turn themselves over and push themselves up. In fact, many of these fundamental exercises tap into that developmental process. Start with picking up one leg at a time; placing hands on the side you are working can help the abdominals contract to create stability through the torso so that limbs can move with ease around the strong central column of trunk. There are so many ways to refine this movement. Imagine picking the leg up from the back of the leg just below the

buttocks. As the knee comes towards the chest, imagine the top of the leg moving subtly in the opposite direction. Keep some weight on the opposite hip: often the weight of the lifted leg creates some unnecessary torque of the pelvis. Stay curious and, when you are ready for a challenge, lift and lower both legs at the same time but be mindful of the lower back, which you can protect by revisiting earlier work. As the legs lower, the pelvis counterbalances by rolling, zipping up, in the opposite direction.

6. The foot is pivotal for walking and standing and deserves special treatment. Extend one leg out to 45 degrees, draw the legs together, and begin by simply pointing and flexing the foot and ankle. Again, the technical names of these movement (dorsiflex and plantarflex) are less important than feeling and sensing the complex movement of the foot. The simple ideas that the big toes have their own muscle and the little toes have their own muscles and that there's a third that connects to the top of the foot helps really flex the ankle fully, which in turn widens the ankle bones. We need strong ankle flexors when we walk—imagine the heel striking softly and then rolling through the foot. Full ankle circles are also a great way to strengthen the muscles all around the circumference of those joints.

7. Lying on the stomach is a crucial part of this fundamental work. To start, lie prone with hands stacked and forward, your forehead resting on the hands. Let the upper chest spread into the mat, because this will help to lengthen the upper back, which tends to round forward slightly. Spend time visualizing the front of the body elongating: stretch the sternum forward, lengthen everything underneath the sternum forward, lungs

324

and heart forward, and keep spreading the chest into the mat. This is also a great place to focus on breathing. Remember there's no one right way to breathe, but try sending the breath into the back of the lowest set of ribs where the kidneys and adrenal glands are located. When ready, try lifting the head, hands and elbows just barely off the mat, extending the upper back. Bend back between the shoulder blades, behind the lungs and the heart. A couple of degrees of movement will train those spinal extensors to support us better when we're sitting and standing. Before moving on, try lifting one leg at a time followed by bending one knee at a time

8. Quadruped position is commonly referred to as "all fours" and is a great strength building position. If knees are sensitive, padding helps. If wrists are sensitive, try making a fist and placing the knuckles on the ground, which stacks the wrist nicely. Start with a simple cat/ cow—flexing and extending the spine. Then find a neutral pelvis: back of the pelvis level with the floor and ceiling. There are so many movement possibilities to explore here. Try shifting the spine forward and backward in space. Simple stability exercises are all challenging progressions, as for example lifting up one limb up at a time, taking opposite arm and leg off at the same time and reaching in opposite directions, adding a small tricep push-up, and eventually floating both knees off the ground together. Making this part of your exercise routine will yield benefits over many years.

9. To finish standing after all the work above is really to recapitulate one's developmental process. Standing well is an art in and of itself that's worth studying and practicing. Start by thinking about the width of your stance. Try standing with the heels

lined up with the sitting bones and the knees lined up with your hip joints. Distribute the weight across the sole of the foot, half the weight in the heel and half the weight in the front of the foot. Make sure you have weight balanced from left to right. Now that the front of the pelvis is level with the wall in front of you, lift the pubic bone up in the front and lengthen the tailbone down to a spot just behind your heels in the back. Elongate your spine by reaching up through the crown of the head and continue to breathe deeply. Adding some additional spinal mobility here can be a way to ensure that the spine has been moved in all directions. Place hands behind the head, look up towards the ceiling with the center of the chest for some spinal extension, and bend sideways for some lateral flexion, rotating right-to-left. Keep the movement controlled and work safely in the mid-range.

Now that you have some fundamentals, including moving the spine in all three planes if safe, you may be ready to start doing some of the beginning Pilates exercises. But remember that these restorative movements are also key to the most challenging exercises. For each of the exercises listed above, there are deeper, more nuanced ways of understanding the exercises, which is why working one-on- one with a trained practitioner is so vital whenever possible. Pair some of the pre-Pilates exercises with some of the cues from the rest position. For example, allow the shoulder girdle (collarbone, upper arm, and shoulder blade) to float up and elevate on the inhale while standing: fill up the lungs more efficiently by expanding the ribcage.

Basics of Breathing

Before we dive any deeper into the Pilates mat repertoire, let's circle back to the breathing since Joseph Pilates said, "Above all, focus on the breath." Remember, there is certainly no one right way to breathe—but there are many ways to play with and explore the breath that can be beneficial.

This can be done pragmatically and doesn't require any metaphysical overlay. For example, practice drawing air in through the nostrils and visualize the air swirling or spiraling in. The nasal passageway is ridged and curved so the air doesn't travel in a straight line. Rather, it is filtered and warmed as it travels through the bronchial passageways. Simply noticing that the air entering the body is cooler than the air leaving the body can be a powerful tool.

Remembering that the oxygen enters the bloodstream on that particular breath is another simple way to deepen the breathing. Just as the ribcage expands on the inhale, imagine all your branches (bronchial and arterial) expanding and dilating on the inhale to allow for more flow.

Perhaps the image of the heart beating slightly faster on the inhale and slowing down gently on the exhale, what's called vagal tone, will enhance our experience of breath here too.

Ultimately, the focus on the breath becomes centered on the diaphragm— our primary breathing apparatus and arguably the most important muscle in the body. The dome-shaped muscle located within the lower portion of the ribcage— underneath the lungs and the heart—contracts and shortens on the inhale; it literally works to create a vacuum pump to help suction air down into the lungs. The feeling of breath moving into the abdomen and the upper chest simultaneously is a powerful indicator of how effectively we are breathing.

In traditional Pilates, a vast majority of the movements are initiated on the inhale. Because Pilates uses body-weight and spring resistance there's generally less compressive load on the supporting structures of the body. We are rarely lifting static weight overhead or in a manner in which that weight would bear down on the body. In those cases, initiating movement on the exhale makes better sense because the abdominal muscles create a better brace on the exhale so that you can "power-lift" the weight up. Pilates is not weight-lifting in the traditional sense but can reinforce and help clarify certain instruction when looked at closely.

In other words, don't adhere to rules alone, but look deeper for the underlying reasons.

Here are three simple ways to reinforce moving on the inhale—as a way to strengthen the diaphragm in coordination with a variety of movement.

1. In the supine position, press the palms of the hands into the ground on the inhale and slowly decrease the pressure on the exhale. Remind yourself that the arms (triceps and lats) are working in the same way at the same time as the diaphragm: they are working and contracting analogously. Then, take the arms up to the ceiling and pull them down to the floor on the inhale.

2. Now the arms are also moving in the same direction as your diaphragm, modeling or mirroring the movement of the diaphragm inside the body. Furthermore, imagine how the space between the fingertips and the shoulders externally demonstrates how the lungs also expand and contract inside of the chest internally. Revisit hands behind the head to lift the head, shoulders, and chest. This time curl up on the inhale so that the abdominals and the diaphragm, again, start working synchronously; they're contracting together, reinforcing the action of the other. However, it can also be useful to reverse this so that the abdominals and the diaphragm work inversely to each

other. Remember the abdominals can contract and help send the diaphragm back up and under the lower ribs. In this respect, the abdominals are secondary breathing muscles; they help facilitate a deeper or more rapid exhale but they are not fundamental to it. You can certainly breathe functionally without the abdominals' assistance, especially when you are resting and simply breathing diaphragmatically. There are times where it is vital to recruit the abdominals' help, as when lifting weights or in fight-or-flight stress response, but then other times where you may want to reduce their presence from the ever-changing equation. Given that fact, try one more pattern here: curl up and hold the position and take a number of deep breaths. Pay close attention to all the changes, some subtle, and some very apparent as you alternate between the inhale and the exhale with the head lifted.

3. If you were able to lift the head comfortably and would like an additional challenge, try maintaining the position while bringing the knees into the chest, heels together, toes apart, knees lined up with the shoulders. Press the legs straight out to a 45-degree angle on the inhale and pull them back in on the exhale. Now you can put some of the pieces together more fully: imagine the diaphragm contracting and pressing down towards the pelvis on the inhale as you send the legs out. You can even imagine sending the breath down into the toes. As the knees come back in, pull the abdominals in and up, then visualize reeling the knees back in from the abdominals, sending the diaphragm back to its starting place.

Matwork— Approaching the 100

In the traditional Pilates group class, this is often a first exercise, which assumes a great deal of bodily awareness and facility. If an individual has a strong movement background and exercises regularly, this can be a great place to start. Otherwise, private instruction and a methodical exploration of some of the fundamentals listed earlier lead up to this. For anyone who's had trouble lifting the head with the hands behind it, slow down: if you've already found your edge with some of the pre- Pilates exercise, spend more time with them.

Additionally, keep seeking the advice from a trained movement professional and give them time to share their wealth of information. If you continue to experience difficulty, try using a prop or piece of equipment.

For example, place a folded towel underneath the upper back— press down into the towel to lift the head up and see if shifting how you create leverage changes anything. You can use something larger (yoga block, Pilates barrel) as a wedge to keep your back elevated, then adjust with the amount of weight you have resting on the supporting structure. There are so many different tricks, slight adjustments, shifts in perspective that keep us from getting stuck, complacent, or satisfied with the status quo.

Before we look at this quintessential Pilates exercise, assuming you are ready for the challenge, let's try something that may help explain the rationale for having this exercise come so early in the system.

1. Lying with your head on the ground and legs long on the mat, reach the arms back overhead—reach for the wall with fingertips, stretch the heels in the opposite direction—and pull the abdomen taut. As the arms return to the ceiling, allow the weight of the arms to sink down through the back of the

ribcage, connecting lower ribs more deeply to the top of the pelvis.

2. Try the same movement (shoulder flexion and extension) with the head raised. If this strains the neck, stop immediately. Otherwise, see how far back the arms can go without the head and shoulders coming down at all. Generate a commensurate amount of force with the abdominals equal to the weight of the arms going back. It's a cantilever and you want the supporting structure to maintain its integrity, resisting gravity's pull down. Don't let your own arms—or anything for that matter—pull you back or down.

3. Now contrast the arms reaching back to bringing the arms just above the pelvis. Notice how reaching the arms forward past the toes with the fingertips helps hold the position.

4. Set up the position with the arms reaching forward. Start pumping the arms straight up and down with a degree of vigor within a controlled range of six to eight inches. Keep it strong and contained. Emphasize the downward action of the arms at first, connecting to the back of the arms and the upper back and using the strong thrust of the arms forward and down to keep the part of your back on the floor firmly grounded. Inhale for five pumps and exhale for five pumps, keeping an even inhale to exhale ratio. Take 10 breaths, which equals 100 pumps of the arms. It's a sprint and will get the heart beating faster when completed correctly. Pilates has an element of interval training: the heart rate rises and falls moderately over the duration of a session.

5. For an added challenge, when ready, practice lifting one leg at a time or lift both legs a few inches off the ground so that the toes are at eye level.

The Roll-Up

The Roll-Up is a benchmark exercise and is performed exactly as it is aptly named, building on the skills already performed in the previous exercise. The idea here is not to foist the weight of the spine and ribcage off the floor with the neck muscles, which are primarily designed to lift the head and cervical spine up solely when lying supine. In order to get the abdominal muscles engaged, effectively remember the important of leverage. We press something down in order to lift something else up, allowing us to lift up more weight than force we are applying to lift that weight up, a hallmark of bio-mechanical efficiency. There's also a subtler aspect to this: leverage allows us to move where we want to move, bend where we want to bend, extend where we want to extend. For a joint to be healthy it needs to be moved in its full range of motion. With roughly 360 joints in the body, there's so much movement potential that can be actualized to keep all those joints rolling, sliding and gliding.

Here are some basic ways to start building a more functional and effective roll-up.

1. Bring the legs all the way together to create a nice boundary or bolt for the pelvis. Make sure the heels are together to help level the pelvis. Lift the head up and check out the position of the legs to see if they appear aligned. If they are veering off to one side, move them center. Placing your own eyes on your body is an important tool. Don't always take someone else's word for it. We want to learn to trust our own perceptions and pair that with information relayed by the outside observer.

2. Remember how important the weight of the arms was in the 100. Start by reaching the arms back overhead again, enjoying the flexion of the shoulders: the collarbones rolling back, the top of the shoulder blades tilting down towards the floor, the side-body lengthening, the low back spreading long and wide. As we bring the arms up to the ceiling, connect the lower ribs to the top of the pelvis and let the upper back get heavier on the mat; use that leverage to bring the chest up and the head will lift up in response. Try reaching the arms forward and down and keep peeling away from the mat. Come up one vertebra at a time by pressing one vertebra at a time down into the mat, by pressing one set of ribs down into the mat at a time. The ribs roll forward as the vertebrae flex forward. Elongate the back muscles as you come all the way up to sitting, reaching forward for the toes with the fingers and the crown of the head. If you find yourself getting stuck on the way up, resist for now the temptation to toss the head or arms down. Truly be patient and teach yourself to appreciate the hurdles you can't quite get over. The body will thank you in the long run because that's where the additional strength is required. It's also the way to build that strength which won't happen if you cheat it. In other words, we get stronger when we don't bypass the places where our weaknesses are revealed. Coming up part-way with good form is often better than coming up all way with a toss or a jerk. In the traditional Pilates mat work, we roll up half-way on the inhale and the rest of the way on the exhale: one full breath cycle on the way up and one full breath cycle on the way down.

3. If rolling up from the lying down position left you stranded slightly, give yourself permission to rock or lift yourself up so

we can practice rolling down. If you rolled up all the way with good form, congratulations: now it's time to keep working and to find new ways to stay challenged. One of the best ways to better and master rolling up is by rolling down with precision, quality, support, and control. Rolling down is initiated in a reversed manner. If the legs are still glued together, reach through the heels without lifting them off the floor, which would indicate knee hyperextension. Without moving the upper body, send the tailbone toward the heels and start rolling the pelvis back, rolling it under. If you keep moving from the pelvis, the upper body will respond by rolling back slowly. See if you can roll back to the base of the sacrum or the waistband of your apparel, pull the abdominals in, and exhale to come back up. Next time, roll down through the five lumbar and see if you can contact the two lowest sets of ribs in the back to the mat, pull the abdominals in, and exhale to come back up. The lower tips of the shoulder blades are the next landmark we encounter before we attempt to roll all the way down to the back of the head again.

4. Pulling the abdominals in when we lift up the weight of the trunk in these exercises is truly paramount. If we neglect pulling the abdominals in, we tend to overwork the hip flexors. Pulling the abdominals in on the exhale in those key moments means you are fulfilling two good fully functional objectives at once. Sometimes we start tuning out details or language that starts sounding rote. Needing constant reinforcement and real concentration is the knowledge that pulling the abdominals as you lift up the trunk is imperative, that it inhibits the psoas and protects the guts and lower back, which has less skeletal support

and more weight to bear than the vertebra above. Imagining the abdominals as scooped out, hollowed out, concave like a valley, like a crescent, is integral to these exercises. If we are not pulling the abdominals in when we lift up the weight of our trunks, we are simply using the wrong muscles—just because it feels like we are using the abdominals doesn't mean we are truly activating them.

5. If you are having trouble with the roll-up, there's one more helpful trick. Give yourself more support by placing a small pillow between the pelvis and the ribcage. Pressing down into the pillow on the way up reminds you to create leverage at the right moment and gives you a little extra lift, a little bit of a head start or boost. These moments can also be refined on the Pilates equipment. Using the spring-loaded bar on the Cadillac can help people who can't do the exercise on their own and can challenge people with added resistance for those who feel they can roll-up with ease.

Bridging

In my teaching practice, we do the Bridge after the Roll-up to build on the skills and concepts that have already been introduced. Traditionally, one would roll the hips all the way over the head and shoulders, and then roll back down. I think the two are closely related and the one can be substituted for the other to help refine and clarify the movement principles. We'll look at the way to start rolling-over, which is suitable to beginners at the end of the section.

1. The Bridge begins with a clear posterior pelvic tilt from the pre-Pilates work. Start with knees bent, feet firm to the mat, heels lined up with sitting bones and the center of the knees aligned with the hip joints. Notice how if the knees open too wide it

forces the weight onto the outside of the foot (supination), and if the knees narrow together it rolls the foot onto the inside (pronation). We keep the knees tracking over the second and third toes in general to keep the angle of the knees from getting too acute or obtuse. This prevents strain on the knees and distributes the weight more evenly across the surface of the joint. We can even project way ahead and start thinking about how these principles can help in our everyday activities and other kinds of training. This kind of focus can help us refine how we go up and down steps, how we sit and stand, how we do our squats.

2. Just as in the Roll-Up, we bridge sequentially through the spine by creating leverage. To lift the pelvis up, we press our low backs softly down. The low back rolls up as we press our lower ribs down in the middle back. The upper back between the shoulder blades becomes thefoundation as we lift the middle back up. Of course, we are trying to integrate the strength in our arms and legs with our torso. Pressing the arms through the extension of the shoulders all the way down to the palm of the hands and fingertips is satisfying and strengthening. Feet can press down and heels can pull back to engage the hamstrings and lengthen the spine past the feet. Feet can also press down and away from the body to engage differently. It's all fair game in the world of movement if done mindfully, with curiosity. Dogma and rigidity do not help us become more integrated. There's no one right way to do any exercise, but we do aim to adhere to the principles of physics and bio-mechanical efficiency such as we understand them in the moment.

3. Rolling down from the bridge is another reversal. Instead of dropping the hips back down, try keeping the hips lifted as you internally curl the ribs and spine back down. We come down one vertebra at a time by lowering one vertebra at a time back to the mat. Imagine the keys of a piano, playing one note at a time. Make sure you do come all the way down and give the pelvis a chance to release fully into the floor before you come up again. Every aspect of the movement is valuable—no moment is more important than any other. This means we are trying to stay connected through the transitions.

4. The breathing in the Bridge is truly fascinating. Inhaling on the way up is a way to strengthen the diaphragm because it places the resistance on a downhill slope. The simplest way to visualize this is to imagine the muscle pushing something up a hill on the inhale, where there's more weight to lift. Rolling down of the exhale helps us contract the abdominals as we try to keep our hips lifted and curl the chest forward internally without lifting the head up.

5. Once you are ready to progress, try rolling your hips off the mat with your feet off the ground, knees bent into the chest. It requires a tremendous amount of effort in the arms. Eventually, we come all the way up to the spread of upper back between the shoulder blades— always being careful not to place too much weight on the back of the head and neck.

Single Leg Circles

Like many Pilates exercises, the single leg circle is a variation on a theme and is linked to the pre-Pilates movement fundamentals. After doing some version of the roll-up and some version of rolling over (bridging), the spine is stabilized again after being mobilized, and we begin to explore the movement in the hip joint again, moving the lower limbs around a strong and steady spinal column.

1. Before circling an extended leg, start in the constructive rest position and place one hand on the hip, reminding it to stay in place, to stay evenly weighted with the opposite hip. Then practice lowering and lifting the knee laterally, foot grounded without any attendant movement in the pelvis. At times, we want to ensure that the movement of our limbs does not destabilize other parts of the body. Later, we will explore integrating fuller movements consciously with sufficient underlying muscular support.

2. Limbering up can always be helpful before doing larger motor movements. Draw one leg in and place the hands behind the hamstrings. Extend and bend the knee with a real sense of ease. Enjoy how the two conjoined sockets of the tibia can glide and slide around the two conjoined balls at the bottom of the femur. Try this with the head and chest lifted. If you find it easier to stretch the back of the leg with the abdominals engaged, we start to become aware of how the body's reflexes, here reciprocal inhibition, help us move more freely. Remember, if you spend a significant amount of time on one side, it is always helpful to pause and feel the consequences of our actions; taking a moment to appreciate the effects of what we've done is a way to maintain those benefits. In other words, we want our sessions to have a lasting impact on our biomechanics and our biochemistry.

3. Single leg circles sometimes seems like a bit of a misnomer: sometimes the movement is more elliptical, D-shaped. We can circumduct our legs through fuller ranges of motion as we get more agile, or reign it in and find the strength in the mid-range. Circling with the leg at a 45- degree angle can be beneficial for people who are tighter. The farther away from center, the heavier the leg becomes relatively, like carrying your grocery bags with the arms out in front compared to letting the arms hang at one's side. Factoring in how gravity is at play in each exercise can yield powerful results. Exploring a range of movement in a safe and balanced way within the relative constraints of a certain exercise is another way of building strength and body awareness.

4. Eventually the movement of the limbs, pelvis, and trunk becomes more integrated. Returning to the CRP, try rotating the pelvis subtly side-to- side, alternating where the weight is placed on the back of the pelvis, moving the pelvis side-to-side like a see-saw, and allowing the knees to move like windshield wipers. For added challenge, try the same movement with the knees up in a tabletop position; add a circular motion of the pelvis and imagine you are moving through all the numbers of a clock face or all the points of a compass. Eventually, one leg extends out long on the mat, and with the knee bent or extended the entire spine rotates over into a supine twist.

Rolling Like a Ball Preparation

1. Transitions to come up to sitting by rolling up, rocking up, or turning to the side all work well. The next exercises capitalize on a number of our fundamentals, including pelvic tilts and breathing. From a seated position, knees bent, feet on the floor,

hands behind hamstrings, practice rolling back a quarter of the way, perhaps to the base of the sacrum and coming back up. Initiate from the pelvis on the way down by tilting the hips back intentionally from the lower aspect of the abdominals. Return by hugging the abdominals together and exhaling fully. It's worth my repeating that pulling the abdominals drawn together, in and up as you lift the weight of the trunk back up, is functional on two-levels: it inhibits the hip flexors from doing the work that the abdominals are better suited for, and it is aligned with proper breathing mechanics. We don't trust our feelings on this. Rather, we trust our intellect, interrogating ourselves and the movement for maximum gain: are we really drawing the abdominals in when we lift up the weight of our trunks? This is imperative: it protects the spine, the organs, and helps us breathe more efficiently.

2. Try the same exercise with the feet lifted just off the mat. Start with the hands behind the hamstrings and eventually place the hands on the front of the shins. Visualize the spine growing taller over and around the knees. See the armpits rising over the knees or be extravagant and see the lower ribs in the front rising over the knees. Sometimes we imagine the impossible to find out what is possible. Pelvic tilts with the feet lifted will start to rock the body back. How far back can you rock without tipping all the way over and rolling all the way back? Hone in on the moment of initiation. Keep pulling the abdominals in when needed and pairing that engagement with the breathing.

3. One other way to feel the power of this suggestively embryonic shape is to return to the back and practice lifting the head and tail off the mat simultaneously, especially if the spine is known

to be healthy. Try placing the hands behind the head and lifting the head and feet at the same time, bringing the knees to the elbows at the same time that you bring the elbows to the knees. This position engages the abdominals fully, from top-to-bottom and bottom-to-top. If there are concerns about spinal health, this movement can be performed lying on the side with a much smaller range of motion.

Series of Five

Pilates exercises tend to get more challenging. They follow a pattern of moving up a ladder. Generally, the exercises get progressively more difficult through the workout. Regressions—doing easier or modified versions—can also be seen as helping us work harder. Giving oneself a spot or assistant, for example, should deepen the work rather than allowing a way to skip over or bypass a tough spot.

1. One example of giving ourselves a helping hand also teaches us how to use our own body as a better training partner. Draw one leg into the chest and place the hands on top of the shin. Then, press the shin up into the hands, pull the hands down into the shin, pull the knee into your chest with your arms, and press the leg away from the chest just as strongly. Find just the right amalgam of push and pull here, and then feel the body working together. Try lifting the head up and notice how the arms, the abdominals, and the leg all conspire to help you stay up— we're stronger when we use the body in a unified way, finding the gestalt, the totality greater than the sum of its parts.

2. When ready, lift the opposite leg off the ground and slowly switch from side-to-side. Playing with the tempo, sometimes slower and sometimes at a quicker pace, is another way to keep

building dynamic strength. We never want the movement to become pat or routine.

3. Eventually, we progress to taking both legs out for a double-leg stretch; move to straight leg scissors with the hands placed behind the leg or ankle. Practice double-leg lower lift with the hands behind the head, and criss-cross right elbow to left knee with right leg outstretched to the other side, then left elbow to right knee with left leg outstretched to the other side.

4. Variations of the exercises above include doing the entire series with the hands behind the head, or with hands or even a pillow placed underneath the back of the pelvis. The sky's the limit when it comes to doing the Pilates exercises, and this is just an introduction to the breadth of movement possibilities we aim to consider, the wide-range of movement patterns we hope to explore. For the more advanced practitioner, weights and other forms of resistance, including industrial-grade springs, add increasing levels of complexity and challenge. Pilates should not overextend or overexert the body but instead should take it right to the edge of what can be done with good form.

5. Before the end of the workout, coming back to a standing posture is generally a good idea. Additional ways of ending might include a set of calf-raises, further exploration of spinal mobility (flexion, extension, side-bending and rotation), and perhaps some standing roll-downs.

Pilates is a time-tested method that continues to evolve. It serves to help us become stronger and more aware in our bodies and can be a container for exploring all manner of biomechanics. It is motivational— it teaches us to hold our ground, stay calm, and work through myriad challenges. It also pairs well with all other activities we aim to achieve: it supplements rather than supplants. Pilates has a rich history with a host of colorful and diverse characters. It truly is a vast system. Individual teachers are the lifeblood or Pilates; much of what is learned and taught is done orally and in-person. At best it isn't scripted or formulaic but discursive and responsive, intuitive and analytic. In short, it must be lived, felt, and experienced.

CONCLUSION, with SUMMARY REVIEW and Motion & Exercise + Workout Plans

Alex Cooksey

When I meet people and introduce myself as a personal trainer, quite often I'm met with innocuous questions like "How should I work out?" or "What should I eat?" I'm sure I annoy people when I reply with the classic, go-to response: "It depends." Admittedly "It depends" is, on its own, a pretty useless answer. We need more context. Some people are interested in the discussion that follows, as I hope you are. For better or worse, there is no one-size-fits-all approach.

This chapter will focus on two primary objectives. First, we will explore the process of setting clear and measurable goals that align with your values and direct you to action. We will also start to examine how your goals should guide your approach to training, nutrition, and other lifestyle decisions.

As nutrition, sleep, stress management, and other essential aspects of healthy living have been examined at length earlier in this book, we then will pivot to a more focused discussion of human movement and exercise.

While we cannot pretend to provide a detailed understanding of these topics here, you should nonetheless conclude this chapter empowered; armed with a practical understanding of exercise fundamentals, you should feel confident to assess and revise your existing training routine as needed, or begin a holistic training routine that serves your needs as well as your goals.

At the very least, you should feel well equipped to know what to look for if you choose to seek professional guidance and coaching.

PART 1: CLARITY IN THE GOAL SETTING PROCESS

OUTCOME GOALS

After you've asked "How should I work out" or something to that effect, and I've told you "It depends" (and you either visibly roll your eyes or just do so in your mind), the first thing we need to explore is your goal.

What do you want? I'm going to have a hard time providing a map and directions if you don't know where you'd like to go.

When most people set health and fitness goals, they think about a desired outcome, a result they'd like to achieve. Often, these results are objective and easily quantified: get stronger, lower blood pressure, lose weight. Other times, the outcome is a bit more fuzzy or subjective: feel more confident, feel more comfortable playing golf, have more energy. Either way is fine—not all things that matter are easily measured.

Most important is that we have a guiding compass so that you're not spending your effort inefficiently, working hard while moving in the wrong direction. That said, even if your goal is more qualitative in nature, it is useful to establish clarity and specificity. After you decide what you want in broad terms, we can translate your goal in such a way that we can more easily assess progress over time. One such method is to develop a SMART goal. SMART is simply an acronym that stands for Specific, Measurable, Attainable, Relevant, and Time Bound.

Specific: This is the overarching umbrella—think who, what, when, where, why, and how. If your goal is to lose weight—how much? By

when would you like to lose it? Are there any other parameters or conditions that you'd like to meet while losing the weight? You want to be
muscular...so, like Arnold Schwarzenegger? Or are we just talking
about filling out a medium size T-shirt instead of a small? Even though
we probably share some thoughts on what it means to be healthy, fit,
or lean, I want to know what exactly that means in your head. If your
goal is to have more energy or feel more confident, think of concrete
examples of what that would look like in your life. Tell me what your
goal means to you.

Measurable: Again, how do you know if you've achieved your goal, or
at the very least are making progress? "Get in better shape" is hard to
measure, and doesn't tell me nearly as much about what you want as
"lose body fat" or "improve cardiovascular endurance." Certain goals,
of course, are harder to quantify—an example earlier referenced, "feel
more comfortable playing golf," can be very difficult to judge objectively, since you're probably evaluating highly subjective feelings like
muscular tension, energy levels, or pain. In cases like these, you can still
come up with proxy measurements that help you understand if you're
making progress.

Maybe this is your score at the end of a round of 18 holes, or just
feeling like you don't need to pop an Advil while you play.

Attainable: Wouldn't it be wonderful if Amazon Prime two-day ship-
ping applied to our health and fitness goals? For many of us, there's a
Goldilocks effect at play when we set goals; something that feels too
easily achieved may not be sufficiently motivating, while too much ambition increases the risk of failure (or compels you to adopt strategies
that may not be in your best interest). Are you hoping in two weeks to

swim the English Channel, but don't currently know how to swim? Maybe your goal for the next two weeks is just to buy a swimsuit, find a nearby pool, and sign up for lessons! When in doubt, start small, especially if you've struggled with your goal in the past. Sometimes the most important part of this whole game is to continually experience the feeling of success and develop a sense of self-efficacy. With long-term goals, by all means you can and should have ambitious goals, but in plotting out your map to victory it's essential to create reasonable expectations. Dream big, but make your way there one step at a time.

Relevant: At surface level, you can simply judge whether your goal connects with something broader that you're working toward. Perhaps you tell me your specific training goal is to increase your one rep max (the most weight you can lift one time) in the bench press. That's great if you're a powerlifter! If your broader goal is to lose fat, a higher one-repmax in the bench press might not be particularly relevant, since you can get a lot stronger without much change to how much muscle or body fat you have. Something like a 10-rep-max in the bench press or the time it takes you to row 2,000 meters would likely be more relevant, from a training perspective.

At a deeper level, it's important to consider whether or not your goal fundamentally connects and resonates with your values and priorities in life. Perhaps you associate gaining muscle with increased confidence, and in turn you associate higher confidence with performing well at your job. Ask yourself whether or not your health and fitness goals really connect with what you want in your life. We all know people who have a six-pack and are still insecure about their appearance. Take the time to consider what really matters to you. The more deeply your health and fitness pursuits connect to your most important values and priorities in life, the easier it will be to do the work necessary to accomplish your goal.

Time-Bound: Simply put, we're putting a deadline on your goal. It's not always critical to achieve our goals by a specific moment in time, and we rarely (probably never) have full control over whether or not we succeed. If you're looking to decrease your blood pressure from 150/95 to 110/70 in 6 months' time, but in actuality "only" lower it to 126/82, I sincerely hope you'll still be proud of the work you put in and happy with what that suggests about your improved health status! It may feel like cognitive dissonance to insist on deadlines without always taking them too seriously. The importance of deadlines is that they promote action and dictate the intensity. You might not have ever taken the steps to lower your blood pressure if it was just something you wanted to achieve "someday."

It's okay to occasionally create your own arbitrary deadlines (many of us do this naturally, anyway—birthdays, trips to the beach, competitions and races, etc.). It's easier to procrastinate and "start next week" when there's no pressure to do the work now, and there's a massive difference in how you'll approach your training, nutrition, and other lifestyle elements if your deadline sits one month away as opposed to one year.

DIFFERENTIATING HEALTH, FITNESS, AND BODY COMPOSITION

Let's revisit the idea of creating relevant outcome goals. Exactly what is it you'd like to improve—health, fitness (aka performance), or body composition, or some combination of the three? Let's explore some definitions.

Health deals with both the quality and duration of your life. In truth, thanks to the blessings of modern medicine, plenty of people live long lives without being particularly healthy. Heck, you can meet most of life's basic needs at the tips of your thumbs on a smartphone. Humans are one of few (possibly the only) creatures for whom physical activity is more or less optional. You don't see cheetahs ordering their meals on Seamless. Realistically, the types of things we can do to promote a state of good health—staying physically fit, maintaining a healthy bodyweight, getting adequate sleep, etc.—will probably help you live longer, all things being equal; however, with respect to longevity, these elements are necessary but insufficient.

To live a long life, go to your doctor's appointments, get your bloodwork done, and be on the lookout for major red flags. Running marathons and drinking kale smoothies can't do much for you if you're living with undetected tumors. Learn your family history and control what you can. Other than that, wear your seatbelt, look both ways before you cross the street, don't smoke, and try to avoid deliberately engaging in stupid or dangerous activities (basically, don't act like a college-aged undergrad). Be careful not to slip and fall in the shower or when walking on an icy sidewalk. Try not to get stuck by lightning. Yes, luck matters. When it comes to longevity, good genetics go a long way, too. Choose your parents wisely.

To achieve a high degree of health and prolong your healthspan, we might start to branch out and think of things like eating enough vegetables, getting plenty of sleep, and training an appropriate amount (we'll speak more on exercise from a health perspective later in the chapter). That said, please consider health beyond the purely physical. Paying attention to your nutrition, sleep, and movement can do amazing things for your cognitive and psychological health as well as your physical well-being; just be careful of extremes. Spending more time at the gym than you do with your family? Forgoing a dinner invitation with friends so you can adhere to a diet best suited to a professional bodybuilder? From the standpoint of your mental and emotional health, you might be better off reading Harry Potter with your kids or grabbing a beer with an old friend (or water, whatever floats your boat). By all means, eat well, sleep, and exercise, but also go take a long walk in nature, from time to time. Mindfully spend time with loved ones and in contemplation. Strive to be a lifelong learner. Dedicate time and energy to work that fulfills you and allows you to wake up each day with a sense of purpose. Practice compassion and forgiveness toward yourself and others. Give back. Be grateful. Find opportunities to laugh and to play. As they say, it's not the years in your life but the life in your years.

Fitness—aka performance—deals with your ability to perform a given task. Achievement at the highest levels of sport isn't always healthy (true for some activities more than others). Becoming a professional football player likely means multiple joint surgeries, chronic pain, and some amount of brain trauma. Even disregarding the injury potential, becoming a champion wrestler or gymnast often involves manipulations of bodyweight that risk acute dehydration and, over time, may result in eating disorders and metabolic disregulation.

Fitness is relative to the task at hand. Being fit as a powerlifter means being able to squat, bench press, and deadlift heavy weights for 1 repetition at a time; who cares if a tortoise beats a powerlifter in a foot race?

An elite distance runner may not be your best bet if you're looking for someone with tremendous upper body strength. The next time you crack open a fitness magazine and get tempted to follow a training program meant for Navy SEALS, ask whether or not you really need to perform at their level in your daily life.

Most of us don't. Most of us can approach fitness as you would an undergraduate college education. Pick a major! Find something you like and get...decent at it. In the meantime, take courses in other subjects to create a broad base of knowledge, thereby avoiding major gaps as well as providing personal enrichment. Major in swimming, but take some classes in Pilates and kettlebell-based strength training. Major in powerlifting, but take some classes in yoga and modern dance. Major in running, but take some classes in rock climbing and Brazilian jiu-jitsu. The world is your oyster. Amateur athletics, should you choose to get more serious, resemble a master's program; professional athletics, a Ph.D. The deeper you go, the narrower your focus becomes. Specificity and specialization come at a cost. When your personal definition of fitness relates to navigating daily life with ease, variability is generally preferable. More breadth, less depth.

Another aspect of fitness, body composition deals with relative amounts of body fat and lean body mass. Aesthetic goals, focused on changing physical appearance by reducing body fat and/or adding muscle, certainly fall under this umbrella. Many measures of physical health (and, depending on the context, fitness) also improve when relatively lower levels of body fat and adequate lean body mass are maintained (approximately 8-20% body fat for men, 16-30% for women). However, changing body composition certainly does not always overlap with health. Elite bodybuilders, particularly near competition, achieve incredibly low levels of body fat while maximizing muscularity... and, by the time they're onstage to compete, often feel terrible. Women who reduce body fat past a certain level can lose their period. A lineman in

American football might deliberately add substantial weight (both muscle and body fat) to become a more effective human wall on the field of play, but nobody said that this will benefit their long- term physical well-being.

Where do you fall in the Venn diagram? There isn't a right answer, truly. What you value and prioritize is for you to choose, and you alone.

What's most important is that you have clarity with where you land and that your behaviors (e.g. training, nutrition, etc.) align with your goals.

Nobody said you're permanently stuck in one spot on the Venn diagram for all time. When I was younger, I, like many young men, cared mainly about the circumference of my biceps and how much I could bench press. Meeting and marrying the woman I love did a lot to dissociate my confidence from what I saw in the mirror or how much weight I could lift. As I write this, I'm training to run a marathon. Cardiovascular training carries myriad benefits for physical well-being, but if long-term health were my sole concern, I'm sure I could get away with far less.

When I was a kid, I reliably got bronchitis and generally detested cardiovascular exercise; when I heard about people running a marathon, I was quite certain it was something I was incapable of. I'm training to overcome a perceived limit I once imposed on myself. I imagine that, after I've finished that last mile, I'll scale back the running substantially. Most of us, as we get older and wiser, think more about the consequences of our actions, both immediate and enduring (hopefully!). We think about training, eating, and living in a way that is sustainable and supports long-term well-being. Nonetheless, it's nice to take on challenges every now and then.

When it's all said and done, almost all the clients I've worked with—almost all people I know—land somewhere in that middle area of the Venn diagram where the three circles overlap. Common sense suggests that health, fitness, and body composition usually overlap, especially for the general public. Maintaining a certain degree of fitness improves your quality of life and can potentially increase your longevity. Eating a "healthy" diet, based mostly on fiber-rich fruits and vegetables, lean proteins, whole grains, and beneficial fats, will likely make it easier to achieve a relatively lean physique. It's true that you can lose weight eating nothing but candy and fast food, but I'll bet that process is a lot easier eating the "healthy" foods previously mentioned … and, over time, your bloodwork will likely look a lot better, too. Thankfully, that Venn middle region is also pretty darned big. Below is a list of basic behaviors I believe fall in that middle realm and serve as a good foundation for most people, most of the time:

- Consume an adequate amount of protein (0.5-1.0g/lb body-weight)
- Eat a wide variety of colorful fruits, fibrous vegetables, starches, grains, and healthy fats, in appropriate quantities for your goals
- Walk 10,000+ steps daily
- Spend time outdoors, in nature if possible
- Sleep 7 hours nightly, more if needed
- Find a form of exercise you enjoy and do it 3-5 days weekly for 30+ minutes, with 2-3 sessions breaking a sweat. Try to include some form of resistance training at least 2x weekly
- Manage physical and psychological stresses

PROCESS & BEHAVIOR GOALS

Once you've established a clear sense of what you'd like to achieve, we dig into the real work of determining how you'll achieve it. In many cases, people actually know enough about what to do. Where most people need help is in figuring out how to consistently perform the basic behaviors, habits, and routines that will help them get there. Want to get more flexible? Stretch. Want to improve your cardiovascular fitness? Go run.

Don't like running? Pick a cardio machine at the gym—no, I don't care which one. Want to lose weight? Be more physically active and try eating more lean protein and vegetables. Want to have more energy? Turn off Netflix and go to bed; I'm guessing you've watched that episode of "The Office" at least 5 times already anyway.

I didn't say anything too revelatory there, right? Obviously there's a lot more nuance to nutrition, sleep, exercise, and most other elements of health and wellness (presumably that's why you're reading this book), but the basics will get you pretty far most of the time. We all know it's good to drink water...so, how much have you had so far today? If you're like most people I know, not that much! Your outcome goal isn't a verb.

Losing weight isn't a behavior, it's a result. You don't just magically build muscles by showing up at a gym; you lift weights, eat sufficient calories, and get enough sleep. What we need is to bridge the gap between knowledge and action.

Take your outcome goal—the thing you really want to achieve. From there, make a list of basic behaviors that you believe will help you achieve it. Some of these might be one-time actions, but most of them will likely be ongoing habits. Author and kettlebell specialist Pat Flynn ingeniously refers to such lists as "Pirate Maps"—follow the steps to get to the buried treasure. To offer a slight alternative, I'd like you to think of your list as a "behavior menu." Here's an example behavior menu I might use with a client whose primary goal is to lose fat (note the deliberate overlap from the list shown earlier):

- Consume adequate protein (~1.0g/lb bodyweight)
- Consume lots of water and vegetables throughout the day
- Focus on eating slowly and thoroughly chewing your food
- Walk 10,000+ steps daily
- 2 or more days weekly resistance training, additional cardiovascular training if needed
- Sleep 7+ hours nightly
- Manage physical & psychological stresses
- Create an environment conducive to fat loss behaviors
- Seek support from your community (family, friends, coworkers, etc)

Though I'd guess you know enough to get started (and our good friend Google is right there at your fingertips), seek expert guidance if you're unsure what basic behaviors will help you make progress!

Once you've created your list, begin by identifying areas you're executing at a high level and on a consistent basis. There's nothing wrong with making further improvements in these areas, but you'll probably see a greater return by investing your efforts elsewhere. From there, we can examine those other areas where you have more of an opportunity to improve. Among this latter group, pick 1-2 areas where you are both interested in making a change and feel capable of doing so.

Maybe you understand sleep is important for recovery, but have a newborn child and feel that improving sleep would be really difficult right now. That's okay! You can still facilitate recovery by working on other habits such as incorporating meditation or doing five minutes of stretching every day. Interested in working on your diet, but really hate the idea of adding more vegetables? If adding more protein sounds more appealing, let's do that right now and worry about the vegetables later!

Rome wasn't built in a day and you don't need to overhaul your whole life right away to make progress. In fact, I'd discourage it. People often underestimate the positive cascade of benefits that can come from small changes (e.g. even if you only explicitly focus on getting more sleep, you might find you have more energy in your workouts, have more mental bandwidth to eat healthier foods, or feel less stressed because you're more productive at work).

Once you've made your menu selection, it's up to you to think about the specific actions you'll take to get it done. There aren't any right answers here; this is where you have to find options that make sense for your unique life circumstances. You want to add more protein? Awesome!

What type of protein will you consume? During which meal?

How much will you add? Adding more protein might include adding a protein shake post-workout, snacking on hard-boiled eggs instead of potato chips, or ordering extra chicken in the salad you get every day for lunch.

Now, let's scale your new habit. Determine how much and how often. Let's say you currently drink an average of 32 ounces of water each day and would like, over time, to increase to 96 ounces. You don't need to immediately adopt a goal of drinking 96 ounces of water seven days a week. You might, for example, set a goal of drinking 48 ounces of water Monday through Friday. How will you accomplish this? By two glasses of water each day, one at breakfast, one at lunch.

Part of the scaling process is also considering potential obstacles and developing contingency plans. Returning to the water example, let's say your tactic to drink more water is to bring a water bottle in to work and keep it at your desk. What do you do if you forget to bring the water bottle one day? What will you do in order to stay on track? Other possible obstacles might simply involve specific actions you need to take to execute your habit. Maybe this is as simple as buying a water bottle if you don't have one yet or setting recurring calendar reminders to drink your water if you're not confident you'll remember.

Give yourself a high chance of success! When scaling your habit, give yourself a target that feels substantial enough to make an impact while remaining conservative and realistic. You should be at least 9/10 confident that you can execute your habit of choice—I guarantee things will come up that you don't expect. Many people get derailed by setting unreasonably high expectations for themselves and then, feeling as if they failed, quit when they are unable to live up to them. The all-or-nothing approach too often results in nothing.

Let's imagine you haven't worked out in years and now set a goal to suddenly begin working out seven days a week (sound like a familiar New Year's resolution?). If, over the next month, you exercise four days a week, you score a 57%. That's a failing grade. If, on the other hand, you give yourself a far more reasonable goal of working out twice a week and consistently go four times, you doubled your goal. Same outcome, very different emotional response. Go celebrate being a rockstar! It may sound cheesy, but understand this crucial point: you are not celebrating working out four times a week; plenty of people do that already. You're celebrating honoring a commitment that you made to yourself in service of a goal you really care about. That is big. Setting small goals doesn't mean you're not allowed to do more, it just means you give yourself a legitimate chance at feeling success.

After a couple weeks (or some other pre-determined amount of time) of working on your new habit, reassess. You should evaluate your progress with both quantitative metrics (like your weight, body fat percentage, or strength) as well as qualitative metrics like your mood, energy, quality of sleep, etc. While it's next to impossible to single out the impact of any given change (assuming your daily life is not so tightly controlled as that of a lab rat), we want to know if the behavior you're working on is making a positive impact in helping you achieve your goal.

The first question to ask yourself is whether or not you were consistent—think 80% or greater execution on your chosen behavior. If you were not consistent, how can we fairly determine if your chosen behavior is moving you closer to achieving your goal? If you were not able to consistently execute your habit, you may consider if it's not the right thing for you to work on right now, or if perhaps you just need to scale it differently for the time being (i.e. lower your target). If you consistently executed the habit, we can then gauge if this is something worth preserving or even expanding. If you enjoyed this new behavior (or at least it didn't make your life miserable) and it seemed to make a positive difference toward your goal, you might keep doing it. On the other hand, if it made no measurable difference (or even if it did but you hated doing it), you might direct your efforts elsewhere.

Ultimately, the whole journey of working toward your goal is simply a process of conducting experiments. Whether you're looking to add a new behavior or reduce/ stop an existing behavior, there's no need to be afraid. You're not making lifelong commitments, you're experimenting to see what feels sustainable, what you like, and what helps you achieve your goals...and what doesn't.

PART 2 HUMAN MOVEMENT AND EXERCISE CONSIDERATIONS

Having explored the process of creating meaningful and specific goals and creating a path of action, we will spend the latter half of this chapter discussing human movement. The aim is to help you identify any critical gaps in your current training routine or to provide an initial direction if you have not exercised consistently for a long period of time. We will consider common types of movements that most people should incorporate into their training as well as different physical qualities that can be developed through the training process. We will finish with some simple but effective examples of how to thoughtfully organize training as well as training considerations to promote successful aging.

FUNDAMENTAL MOVEMENTS

reducti Let's start with fundamental movements, that is, broad types of movement that your body performs on a routine basis, both in the context of structured exercise as well as in daily life. It should be emphasized that we are focusing now on movements, not exercises. When we speak about squatting, for instance, we are talking broadly about a movement in which the hips, knees, and ankles all bend and extend against resistance (generally gravity) while a relatively upright posture is maintained. From the root movement of squatting, we can create countless exercises by manipulating variables such as the equipment used (barbells, kettlebells, bodyweight, machines), how we position the body or external load, and the direction of movement. People who have dealt with injuries and pain in their lower back are sometimes told by doctors or physical therapists to avoid deadlifting (an exercise involving lifting weight from the ground), yet often perform a similar movement when pulling up their pants in the morning or bending over to pick something up off the floor. Deadlifting is an exercise; the "hip hinge" is the movement. A powerlifter performs barbell squats, bench presses, and deadlifts; a yoga practitioner may perform Chair Pose, a Chaturanga Pose, and the Downward Dog Pose. We give these exercises different names, but they are, respectively, the same fundamental movements.

Specific exercise selection may be most directly impacted by the style in which you train (e.g. Pilates vs. CrossFit vs. ice skating) and the equipment you have at your disposal. Exercise selection can also be an important variable to consider if you are dealing with physical constraints related to coordination, strength, mobility, or injuries/pain. A machine bench press might be far more appropriate than a pushup for somebody who has wrist pain. Kettlebell swings involve a motion almost identical to kettlebell deadlifts, but involve a quick and explosive motion; a trainee who cannot perform the kettlebell deadlift proficiently will likely struggle with the coordination and strength required to perform the relatively more advanced swing.

Psychological factors such as confidence and preference are tremendously relevant as well! A lat pulldown may be better than a pull-up for someone who is afraid of falling from the pull-up bar; people who sees themselves as inflexible and clumsy may be highly reluctant to go into a yoga or gymnastics class. It's okay! Don't like running as a way to improve your cardiovascular health? Try the elliptical, rowing machine, or a bicycle instead. Exercises, ultimately, are just tools - a means to an end.

You can't always avoid doing things that are difficult or that you don't enjoy, but you are far more likely to adhere to a training routine that is at least somewhat enjoyable! Unless you participate in a sport that demands you perform specific exercises, make selections that give you the best benefit toward your goal with the least risk and cost.

To speak in greater depth about how to select specific exercises is outside the scope of this book. Rest assured, beginning with relatively simple tools and exercise variations can be a wonderful introduction to improve your movement literacy and physical capability. Any personal trainer or coach worth their salt will perform assessments to help in selecting specific exercises that are most appropriate to you given your training history, preferences, and goals.

Many trainers approach exercise (strength training in particular, perhaps) through the lens of training individual muscles—at times in combination, sometimes in isolation. We ask, "what muscle does this work?" when introduced to a new exercise, and seek to create balance in our training by incorporating sufficient exercise variety to address the entire body. There is nothing wrong with focusing on specific muscles or performing exercises that isolate muscles individually; this is likely the preferred approach for aesthetically focused training (body-building, at the extreme end of this spectrum), and it can be useful when there is a bodemonstrated need to address specific muscles. However, approaching human movement with this mindset sometimes leads us to lose the forest for the trees. In many contexts, it can be helpful instead to think about the types of movement your body performs rather than taking a more narrow focus on particular muscles.

Your body functions as a wonderfully complex and interconnected machine, and viewing exercise through the lens of movement allows us to better appreciate the harmonious nature in which our body coordinates multiple muscles (and, for that matter, other structures and systems like our nervous system or cardiovascular system) to accomplish any given task. The list below of fundamental human movements is by no means all-encompassing, and in daily life we often combine these motions without thinking about it. However, from this simple list we can generate countless exercise possibilities. Perhaps most importantly, you can achieve tremendous efficiency in your training by developing coordination, strength, endurance, and power in these basic movement patterns. Here lies your foundation:

• Upper Body Push:

To paraphrase a definition given by strength coach and author Dan John, upper body pushing movements are those in which you separate yourself from something in your environment. In daily life, this might be pushing a door open or putting a box up on a high shelf. Common exercise examples include push-ups, bench presses, or overhead presses. Broadly speaking, these exercises strengthen the muscles of the chest, shoulders, and triceps (the back of the upper arm).

• Upper Body Pull:

Just as pushing exercises separate your body from something in the environment, pulling exercises draw them together. In daily life, this might be opening the refrigerator door or rowing a paddle on a boat. In the gym, this includes exercises like bicep curls, pull-ups, freestyle swimming or the rowing machine. Pulling exercises are generally used to strengthen muscles of the upper and mid back as well as the biceps (the front of the upper arm) and forearms, contributing to grip strength.

• **Squat/Lunge:**

Sometimes called "knee dominant" movements, squatting and lunging are lower body movements that generally involve a deep bend at your hips, knees, and ankles. You will usually maintain a more upright posture. Many different squat and lunge variations exist, using different foot positions, directions of movement, and equipment. Some machine- based exercises like leg presses can also be included here, since the basic mechanics and muscles involved are largely the same. These movements often rely on muscles of the thigh (especially the quadriceps, in front) and hips to create motion.

• **Hinge:**

These are lower body movements that primarily involve a deep bending and extending of your hips, with relatively less motion at the knees and ankles; for this reason, many people refer to hingeing movements as "hip dominant." While hinge and squat exercises generally share many characteristics, most standing hinge exercises feature a less upright posture.

The most obvious instances of hip hingeing in daily life are present in moments of bending over to pick things up from the ground. Example exercises include deadlifts or kettlebell swings, as well as glute bridges or hip thrusts (which are generally done lying on your back). Like squats and lunges, hinge exercises challenge muscles of the lower body including the thighs (often biasing the hamstrings, in back) and hips.

• Core Stability:

Ask ten different coaches which muscles belong to the "core" and you might well get ten different answers. As before, all the muscles and tissues of the human body function in such an interconnected manner that it is truly difficult to consider the muscles of the midsection in isolation from the rest of the body. Indeed, "core" is kind of a nebulous term, but for our purposes here we are speaking of the area around the midsection, perhaps between the hips and the ribcage. When stable, the core helps transmit force between the upper and lower body.

This doesn't mean the muscles of your midsection (and, with them, your lumbar spine back) shouldn't ever move through their natural range of motion; context matters! A dancer's core can and should move much differently from someone lifting hundreds of pounds; the "core training" that each of these individuals performs may differ substantially as a result.

That said, when we refer to core strength, we can generally think of creating stability in three planes of motion: front-to-back, side-to-side, and in rotation. Stability, as we'll discuss later, is not an absolute lack of movement; it is the capability to prevent unwanted motion.

Front-to-back stability means preventing excess forward and backward bending of your spine. Planks are a simple but useful example of an exercise that develops this type of stability. Side-to-side stability involves preventing your body from tilting sideways (think of walking with a heavy bag of groceries in one hand), and can be developed with exercises like side planks or suitcase carries. Rotational stability involves the prevention of unwanted twisting of your body; it is essential to many sport movements like kicking, throwing, or swinging a club/racket; rotational stability can be developed with many exercises that only involve one arm or one leg working at a time, such as single leg deadlifts or one arm rows, or exercises that rely on opposite arm and leg working together, like crawling.

• Locomotion:

Locomotion broadly refers to transporting your body through space. While any of the fundamental movements listed above can be performed in such a manner, we often perform them in a relatively stationary fashion in the context of structured exercise; locomotion is therefore deserving of separate mention. Walking and running are the most obvious examples; so easily taken for granted, they are incredibly complex motions that involve coordinating all major joint systems of the human body. Blurring the line between general physical activity and exercise, walking deserves particular attention. Special circumstances aside, walking is the lowest hanging fruit to pick for developing general physical fitness, especially for those who have been highly sedentary for many years or have numerous training limitations. While we cannot pretend that walking 10,000 steps a day will prepare you to be an Olympic champion, the benefits (improvements of cardiovascular health and circulation, respiratory health, strength of muscle, bone, and connective tissue, etc.) of general activity are innumerable.

External load can also be added to locomotion with excellent results. Exercises such as suitcase and farmer carries (which involve walking around holding weight in one or both hands, respectively) challenge the strength of one's grip, balance, and postural integrity while moving through space.

• Breathing:

To speak of breath as a fundamental movement may seem obscure, and yet it is the only movement within this list that is truly essential for survival.

Everybody alive breathes; we all participate in the act of drawing in oxygen and expelling carbon dioxide. If you're reading this book, be proud—without question, you're already doing one of the fundamental movements. Good on you!

Among this list of basic movement patterns, breathing is unique in that it can be performed involuntarily (unless you, unlike most of us, are routinely doing squats and bicep curls in your sleep). However, great benefit can be had from bringing conscious attention to how you breathe. By consciously controlling the rate and mechanics of breathing, you can substantially impact both your health as well as physical performance.

Try this experiment: set a timer for 2 minutes; breathe in for 5 seconds through your nose, then out through your mouth for 10 seconds (try 2 in and 4 out if that is difficult). As you breathe in, imagine expanding your belly in 360 degrees like you're filling up a balloon; try to breathe into the waistband of your pants without actively pushing your belly out. As you exhale, allow this balloon to slowly empty as you breathe out as much of your air as possible. After two minutes, relax for a moment before moving on. When ready, set a timer, this time for only 30 seconds (possibly less); this time, breathe in through your nose for one second, and breathe out forcefully your mouth for one second.

While as before you can try to fill your belly as you breathe in and empty it upon the exhalation, you may naturally find your chest expanding and shoulders lifting with the breath.

What differences did you notice during these two experiments? Most will find their heart rate and blood pressure lower (if you're able to measure) after the slower breathing cycle, and may even feel a sense of calm.

The latter method is much more stimulatory, and will likely raise your heart rate. The first is more appropriate as a default manner of breathing throughout the day and can be useful when trying to shift into a more relaxed state, such as when trying to sleep, calm down from a tense situation, or as part of practices like meditation. Yawning in the middle of an important meeting, or getting ready to go do a hard workout? Try some cycles of the faster breathing and see if that doesn't light a fire in you.

MOVEMENT QUALITIES

After considering different fundamental types of movement, we can think about movement qualities. These are basic physical attributes that can be developed across the entire body and expressed through any and all of the different fundamental movements.

• Strength

Physical strength can be broadly thought of as the ability to exert or withstand force, generally in relation to something in your external environment.

While we typically think of using strength to produce motion, it is also essential in the prevention of unwanted motion, which we call stability (more on this in a moment). It should also be noted that, while many of us associate "strength" with maximal strength (e.g., the most weight someone can use for one repetition of an exercise), strength is relative. Increasing the amount of weight you can use for five repetitions signifies an increase in strength just like an increase in a one-rep maximum.

Muscular development and strength increases often go hand-in-hand, but not always. Strength is also highly dependent on the nervous system, as your brain coordinates your body's efforts to maximize force and coordinate your muscular effort in the most efficient manner possible.

Proper alignment is also critical to strength optimization (try holding a two-pound weight overhead as opposed to directly in front of you at shoulder height). Some people shy away from strength training if they are averse to gaining excessive amounts of muscle, but this need not be the case. While building muscle mass can benefit health, performance, and body composition, strength carries its own benefits and can be developed somewhat independently.

Strength is often referred to as the master quality—that is, generally speaking, increasing strength generally allows you more readily or thoroughly to develop the other physical qualities listed here. Put another way by Brett Jones, "Absolute strength is the glass. Everything else is the liquid inside the glass. The bigger the glass, the more of "everything else" you can do. This idea has obvious limits in practice. All of us are limited by both the amount of time we have to train as well as our physical ability to recover from training; past a certain point strength may not be what limits your improvement and time must be spent developing other qualities or refining technique. Otherwise, the strongest among us would also run the fastest, be the most flexible, and perform the best in all athletic endeavors.

What is important to understand is that strength often is a limiting factor in improving your physical well-being. Yes, you might be able to improve your posture with a lot of stretching and foam rolling, but the lowest hanging fruit might be strengthening muscles like those of your upper back, which can help prevent slouching. You can do all the fancy breathing drills you like, but your breathing mechanics will also improve if you strengthen your lungs, diaphragm, and other breathing muscles through consistent cardiovascular exercise.

Generally speaking, strength is optimally developed through multijoint exercises that involve many major muscle groups at once and can be progressively loaded over time. Preferred choices include variations of squats, deadlifts, lunges, bench presses, pull-ups, rows, and loaded carries (e.g., farmers carries and suitcase carries). On a final note, most people don't ever need to test their maximal strength. If your workouts often involve banging your head against the wall to see how much weight you can use for one rep, just know that you can get extremely strong with much less risk. Performing lifts at or very close the limits of your strength is highly fatiguing and carries a greater chance of exceeding what your body can tolerate. Occasionally testing a one-rep max can be highly enjoyable (and, let's be real, stokes the ego), but just know that you can train to a high level of strength at lower intensities, in sets of three to eight reps, give or take.

• **Mobility & Flexibility:**
While these terms are often used interchangeably, and mobility and flexibility are highly related, they have some important differences. Think of mobility as the ability of your individual joints to move through a certain range of motion without external influence. Flexibility refers to the overall ability of a muscle to be lengthened (stretched), with or without external assistance. Mobility can be position specific; some people can lift their arms overhead if lying down on their back, but struggle to do so when standing up. Executing basic strength training exercises through a full range of motion can be a fantastic means of preserving and often improving mobility and flexibility in tandem with

methods such as stretching, massage, and training methods that focus on flexibility development such as yoga.

Though almost all joints of the body have some capacity for mobility, many mobility issues can be addressed by tending to the shoulders, the thoracic spine (the upper part of your spine, in the same approximate range as your ribcage), the hips, and the ankles. Each of these areas is capable of motion in all three planes of motion (front to back, side to side, and rotation); issues can arise if a loss of mobility in these segments results in compensation from other areas of the body. Likewise, a well-balanced training routine should aim to maintain an amount of muscular flexibility appropriate to an individual's needs and goals (a gymnast needs far more hamstring flexibility than a sprinter, or most people for that matter). For those who spend significant amounts of time sitting, I highly encourage regular stretching of the calves, hip flexors (muscles at the front of your hips and thighs, chest, and lats (large muscles that run along your back, terminating near your armpit). These are, of course, generalizations and your individual needs may differ significantly. Find a trainer, physical therapist, or other movement coach properly certified (through systems such as FMS or PRI) to better understand your needs. Whether due to past injuries, sedentary lifestyles, or other realities of getting older, many of us lose mobility and flexibility we took for granted when younger. Do not allow this to prevent you from training!

Not all exercises are appropriate for all people; stick to exercises you are able to perform comfortably and safely with good technique ("perfect" technique does not exist!). Often, you can modify an exercise or your setup to train around any limitations you might have in order to still make progress toward your goals. For example, someone with very little available motion at their ankles will often be very bent over when squatting, which prevents them from training the muscles they intend to target and potentially causes discomfort over time. A barbell back squat (where weight is placed across the upper back) may not be appropriate.

However, by elevating this person's heels and having them hold weight in front of their body, they may be able to squat with their body in a far better position and enjoy the wonderful benefits we typically associate with the squat movement. Always do what you can, where you are, with what you have.

• Coordination:

Coordination is the purposeful combination of movement and force to complete a desired task. Your brain and body are in constant dialogue, with sensory information sent to the brain and movement commands in turn sent out to the body. No different from learning to play an instrument or speak a language, movement can be approached as a skill to be learned and refined over time. Part of training involves strengthening your "hardware"—building up stronger bones and muscles, creating more mobile joints and resilient connective tissues, etc.—and part of it involves upgrading your "software" by learning and practicing progressively more complex movements (don't misinterpret this as encouragement to do the most awkward, convoluted exercises you can think of!). Although we've spoken of a small number of fundamental movements, remember that you can create almost infinite variety of specific exercises to expand your movement literacy over time. Showing up to the gym and trying to do Olympic weightlifting exercises or backflips can be a recipe for failure and humiliation: there's too much going on! Start simple, with exercises that you can confidently execute with clean technique, and build up to more complicated movements depending on the demands of your particular health and fitness goals. Machines can be a wonderful place to begin for many people, providing an opportunity to make progress toward their goals while developing confidence and basic physical capacity. To use a familiar cliche, mastery is generally defined not by the ability to do the complex, but rather by the ability to do the basics at an exceptionally high level.

• Stability & Balance

Stability pertains to the ability to prevent unwanted motion. People too often mistake stability to denote a lack of movement, especially with regard to core training. If you want a lumbar spine that does not move, vertebral fusion is an option, but not recommended unless truly necessary!

Having a stiffened midsection is much more important if you're lifting hundreds of pounds off the ground than if you are lifting a feather. In training, many people struggle to prevent their shoulders from shrugging upward when doing upper body exercises; this doesn't mean the goal is to lock your shoulder down and back at all times. Look in the mirror and try lifting your arm overhead with your shoulder pulled down away from your ear the entire time; compare that to letting your shoulder shrug slightly when reaching your arm up. Which was more comfortable? Stability is not about eliminating motion entirely, it's about having appropriate amounts of movement. Relative to machines, free weights often require more effort to stabilize your body, the equipment, or both. Some equipment further increases these challenges by creating inherent instability or distributing the weight differently—to experience this, try lifting equivalently an equivalently heavy dumbbell, kettlebell, and half- full jug of water.

Balance relates to your body's ability to keep your center of mass over your base of support; more simply, we generally think of balance as your ability to remain upright or otherwise properly oriented for the task at hand (for example, not falling off the side of a bench when lying down to perform a bench press). Maintaining balance requires stability, especially through the midsection and lower body when standing. This entails having adequate strength in the tissues around the feet, ankles, knees, and hips to prevent postural collapse. Balance is also highly neurological, relying on proper coordination and rapid response to direct appropriate changes of body position in the face of disturbance.

• Power

Power introduces a time component to strength. If strength pertains to the ability to either produce force (acceleration) or absorb force (deceleration), power generally denotes the ability to do so quickly. If two people squat one repetition of 200 pounds, but one of them is able to perform the movement more rapidly, that person has demonstrated more power. Running requires more power than walking. Many exercises that are used for the purpose of power training are explosive in nature, and may thus require a greater amount of coordination and tissue resiliency (especially if impact forces are involved). For this reason, power training is generally not recommended for someone who is new to training or has not trained for a substantial period of time.

That said, the ability to express power is essential to almost any sport activity; think of swinging a racket or club, running and changing direction, or throwing a ball. It can also be critical for safety. Your ability to jump to safety or catch yourself and prevent a fall both rely on power (can you jump slowly, or trip and catch yourself slowly?). While absolute strength can be maintained to a surprising degree as we age, power and speed are among the physical qualities lost most rapidly. Wonderful progress can be made simply by performing basic exercises more rapidly at first, and later introducing explosive exercises and those involving impact when and if appropriate. To properly train power, you'll generally perform very few total repetitions and take relatively longer rest periods since the ability to produce maximal power fatigues you quickly. Approach each rep deliberately so as to maximize explosiveness.

• Endurance

While we will touch on cardiovascular health and fitness shortly, here we are referring to muscular endurance, the ability of a muscle (or muscles) to exert force consistently or repeatedly over a period of time. To illustrate the difference, an athlete who has spent many years swimming may have tremendous cardiovascular endurance, but may not have developed adequate muscular endurance in muscles like the calves should they decide to run a marathon on a whim. A powerlifter may be able to bench press more than double their own bodyweight, but it's quite possible they would lose a push-up contest to any number of group fitness devotees. Maximal strength and strength endurance are two different animals. Training muscular endurance can play a critical role in living life comfortably from a physical standpoint, whether that's having the stamina to play with your kids, maintain a good posture with less effort, or go backpacking with your friends and not feel like you need a rest every 30 seconds when going up a steep hill. In an exercise setting, muscular endurance is typically trained with moderate weight, higher repetitions, and shorter rest periods.

Energy Systems Development & Cardiorespiratory Fitness

Entire books are dedicated to speaking about the development of cardiorespiratory fitness and energy systems development; here we will attempt to provide a cursory understanding of their function and importance. Cardiorespiratory fitness relates to the body's capacity to circulate blood among various organs and tissues, delivering oxygen and other essential nutrients while removing metabolic waste products. Energy systems are the mechanisms by which your body creates the necessary energy needed for all bodily function, including but most certainly not limited to movement.

There are three energy systems, or pathways, through which your body can produce energy. The differences between them lie in their relative rates of energy production and capacity to sustain energy production. One system, referred to as the phosphocreatine system, produces energy at the fastest rate but has a limited capacity to do so. This system dominates in efforts of maximal intensity and minimal duration, up to approximately 10 seconds (it is common to see Olympic sprinters slow down even before the end of a 100 meter race!). An example workout might involve 8-10 intervals of 5-10 seconds apiece, with 3-5 minutes of rest between efforts. Possible exercises used might include sprinting, a rowing machine, jump squats, or a stationary bicycle.

The second system, referred to as anaerobic glycolysis or the lactic acid system, can still produce energy at a high rate, though not as high as the ATP-CP system, and can be the dominant pathway in efforts up to 1-2 minutes at high enough intensities. In track and field, the 400 and 800 meter runs are known as particularly brutal events due to the exceptional degree of fatigue and sensation of your lungs, heart, and muscles being on fire! Many CrossFit or high intensity style classes challenge this system. An example training session might involve 4 to 6 intervals of working for 1 minute at a high intensity and resting for 2 minutes.

Finally, and perhaps most familiar, the aerobic system has the slowest rate of energy production but by far the greatest capacity. As your body exerts effort for longer periods of time, your relative ability to produce force necessarily decreases and your body relies increasingly on energy production via the aerobic pathway. Classic examples might include long-distance runs or bike rides of 30 or more minutes at a low intensity, but can also include higher intensity workouts such as 12 to 15 intervals working for 30 seconds and resting for 30 seconds, or 4 to 6 intervals of 2 minutes work and 1 minute rest. In the latter two example, the relatively short recovery period and the high number of intervals dictate that the relative intensity of each interval must be lower and that your body must produce much of its energy aerobically.

It seems that, for a while, aerobic training fell out of favor in the fitness industry while high intensity interval training carried far more appeal (when people suggest that intense 7-minute workouts can deliver the same benefits as a lower intensity, 60-minute workout, it's understandable that many would opt for the 7-minute option). However, the foundation of cardiovascular fitness must be initially built with basic aerobic capacity. While lower intensity, long-duration cardiovascular exercise is likely overrated from a fat loss standpoint, it is enormously beneficial for the health of your heart, lungs, arteries, veins, brain, and nervous system. Moreover, your ability to recover is largely driven by the aerobic system, both during exercise and in between sessions. If you find yourself needing a lot of time to catch your breath between sets of squats, for example, you might find that spending some time improving your aerobic system helps you get more out of your sessions by allowing you to get more done in the same amount of time. This certainly does not mean that you need to become a triathlete if your goal is building muscle, only that cardiovascular strength and endurance do occasionally limit people's capacity to train more effectively.

Even brisk walking can be highly beneficial, but cardiovascular exercise can be as diverse as running, biking, swimming, dance, martial arts, or even just a trusty machine at the gym with a built-in TV to play Netflix for you. For most people, including two to three days of aerobic training (even lasting as briefly as 20 to 30 minutes) will be enormously beneficial and is highly recommended . . . and no, getting your heart rate elevated doing lunges is not the same thing. Many people now have access to heart rate data on their phones, smartwatches, or cardio training equipment at the gym; aerobic work will often involve a slightly lower heart rate, especially for longer intensity workouts (one guideline developed by Phil Maffetone uses a default range of 160 minus your age up to 180 minus your age, with some modifications available based on fitness level). Other options include regulating your effort by breathing in and out only through your nose or by ensuring that you can comfortably hold a conversation in full sentences as you exercise.

No one system ever functions independently of the others; you are never exclusively producing energy through any one pathway. Understanding these different pathways can be essential for directing your training in a manner best aligned with your health and fitness goals.

• Muscle Building and Fat Loss

Muscle development and fat loss may not be physical qualities, per se (both of these can be accomplished in the process of developing other physical qualities), but deserve to be addressed here since they are the desired outcome of many people's training. Many other factors outside of training will dictate muscle development and fat loss (such as eating enough or sufficiently few calories, respectively), but here are some brief training considerations.

Generally speaking, training to build muscle might involve slightly higher repetitions (and, consequently, slightly lower weight) than training purely to increase strength. This relates both to repetitions done in each set, but perhaps more importantly to the number of total repetitions done in a workout or even over the course of an entire training week. For example, performing a squat workout with three sets of five repetitions may be preferable for strength development, while a session of seven sets of five may better stimulate muscle growth. Although many classic training texts recommend sets of approximately six to twelve repetitions to focus on muscle growth (and this is a fine starting point), contemporary research demonstrates muscle being built in repetition ranges as wide as three to 30 repetitions per set, provided adequate intensity.

Most beginner and intermediate trainees would still do well to focus on some of the basic exercises previously discussed. This generally means focusing more on multi-joint exercises that involve many large muscle groups, especially if training time is limited (for example, selecting chin-ups rather than bicep curls, even if you want bigger arms). Incorporating other exercise variations, machines, or isolation movements can be highly useful to address any gaps and increase the total stimulus to your muscles with lower cost on your ability to recover.

Training for fat loss need not include endless hours of cardiovascular training; although exercise will certainly burn calories, your nutrition is far easier to manipulate. Orient your training to maintaining muscle mass so that, as you lose weight, you lose as little lean body mass as possible and maximize fat loss (this also makes it easier to keep the fat off after the fact). As such, training during fat loss will often resemble training to build muscle: the style of training that will optimally stimulate muscle growth during periods of higher calorie intake is, unsurprisingly, the style of training that helps maintain muscle when food intake is decreased. Other minor differences might include incorporating more general physical activity throughout the day (and perhaps a bit more cardiovascular exercise as needed), and you might progress your workouts by taking less rest rather than increasing the weight or repetitions from one week to the next.

PROGRAM ARRANGEMENT

Session Organization

Up to now, we have spent this section of the chapter discussing different training considerations. We'll now turn our attention to laying these components out in a practical manner in the context of a training session. Important components of a typical training session include a warm-up, power and strength work, energy systems development (aka cardio), and the cool-down.

According to chiropractor, physical therapist, and strength coach Charlie Weingroff, a proper warm-up accomplishes four main tasks.

First, the warm-up serves to increase core body temperature—literally, you are warming your body up. Merely body temperature and facilitating blood circulation can immediately improve measures of movement quality such as flexibility, strength, power, and muscle elasticity. Second, the warm-up helps to stimulate the central nervous system. You are preparing your body for the intense neurological demands of training, whether that involves producing high levels of force or coordinating complex movements. Third, warming-up allows you to express your current levels of mobility and flexibility. The goal is not necessarily to increase mobility; you're making sure you have access to what you need in order to perform well in that day's workout (if the goal is to increase range of motion in a movement, prepare to use much less load or force). Finally, the warm-up serves as a dress rehearsal for the main movements of your training session. Simply put, if you are preparing to squat, your warm-up can and should include movements that resemble squatting.

This serves both to help warm-up the specific muscles and tissues involved in the exercises you'll be doing as well as to allow you to practice and refine technique, making any necessary adjustments as necessary before the stakes get higher with more weight, speed, etc. The warm-up period can also serve as an ideal opportunity to work on learning new movement skills. If the goal is to learn or polish technique on a relatively new skill, you will be better served to do this while you are mentally and physically fresh, rather than near the end of a training session when you are exhausted. You can also use this time to do any desired work to improve movement quality (sometimes called "corrective" exercises); these are generally low-intensity drills, sometimes passive, that aim to change movement behavior by increasing joint mobility, muscular flexibility, coordination, or muscular awareness (sometimes called "activation drills").

Both of these are fine things to spend time on; just be wary of dedicating so much attention and time to either of these that you forget to actually train with good effort toward your main goals. If you're working to lose 50 pounds, spending half of your time at the gym on a foam roller just won't cut it. Hips feel tight and deadlifting doesn't feel good that day? Skip the 20 minutes of hip stretches just so you can deadlift, and go do something else instead that doesn't need as much hip mobility. You can stretch your hips that night while you're watching TV and deadlift next time!

After warming up, you'll generally want to prioritize exercises that are more complex, involve a high degree of force production, and involve multiple muscle groups. As such, power exercises will typically come first if they are part of your program. From there, focus on bigger, multi-joint strength exercises, especially those which involve heavier weights in your particular session. A barbell bench press would likely precede a dumbbell bench press due to the greater capacity required to lift heavy weights using the barbell. Pull-ups and bicep curls both tax the muscles that bend the elbow; the pull-ups would likely precede bicep curls, since they involve more muscle groups and are more systemically taxing than the curls. Generally, as you get later into the workout and into a deeper state of fatigue, you can pick exercises that are simpler and create less overall fatigue. While you might still feel as if you're working hard on the leg extension machine in the 50th minute of a one hour workout, the overall challenge on your body is nowhere near what it would be if you were exerting an equal amount of perceived effort on a barbell squat. Loaded carries are another personal favorite—for the most part, I trust myself and my clients to walk with decent technique, even when fatigued.

There are numerous ways to organize and combine different exercises within this main portion of the workout. At times, you will perform one exercise in isolation and rest before performing that same exercise again. In other models, you might combine multiple exercises in a group (often called supersets or circuits depending on how many exercises are included in one group), sometimes working the same muscle group, in other instances working opposing muscle groups. When pure strength is the goal, it can be helpful to train at a relatively slower pace in which you allow yourself plenty of rest. This might look like performing a set of five repetitions in the deadlift with a relatively high weight, then resting 3 minutes before performing the deadlift again. For many people, however, time efficiency is maximized with circuit training where three or four exercises are grouped back-to-back. By combining exercises with relative overlap in the muscle groups used, a greater training density can be achieved while still allowing decent rest for any one muscle group along the way. An example of this would be performing a squat, followed by a push-up, followed by a chin-up, with relatively little rest between the individual exercises. Although it may feel fast-paced, the muscles powering each individual exercise rest while the other two are performed. This style of training can also carry value for fat loss training, where the goal over time may be to perform a greater total amount of work. As per usual, how you choose to structure your workout depends entirely upon your goal as well as practical considerations such as how much time you have available to train. I'm sure this can all get overwhelming, and it can certainly be helpful to seek the help of a coach so that you can just dedicate your mental bandwidth to showing up and working hard, Don't be discouraged! Most any program can work for a while provided you show up and consistently put in a good effort.

After performing the main strength training of your workout, you may consider incorporating energy systems development (cardio training) toward the end of your workout. If your schedule allows, it can often be advantageous to perform cardiovascular work on a separate day from your strength training in order to produce more effort and thus experience greater benefits. However, if it's more practical and realistic to include cardiovascular work during the same session as your strength training, that is totally fine as well. Moreover, most forms of cardiovascular exercise (particularly those done using a machine) will also involve less complicated technique than many strength training exercises, and thus are still suitable to be performed after the rest of training.

Whether or not some form of cardiovascular training has been included, effort should be made to cool down after training. This may include such elements as deep breathing, stretching, foam rolling, using a steam room/sauna, or contrast baths/showers (alternating using heat and cold). Some of these focus on cognitive and psychological relaxation while others focus on physical aspects like promoting circulation. The general concept is to have some way to bring your body and mental state back down to baseline after the stimulation of your training session, thus facilitating the start of the recovery process.

Program Organization and Progression

The difference between merely working out and legitimately training is that training represents a purposeful approach toward exercise that is directed at accomplishing specific goals. By extension, a proper program organizes your individual training sessions in a cohesive manner so that you can make as much progress as possible given the constraints of your time, energy, and ability to recover. Programs commonly last between six to twelve weeks, though shorter and longer options certainly exist; this generally is enough time to allow adaptation while avoiding physical or mental burnout (generally, one or multiple parameters of the program will progress in difficulty as the program goes along, such that the end of the program represents a climax or opportunity to test performance).

Most training programs are organized week-to-week, since most people plan their lives this way naturally. As such, likely the most important factor to consider when laying out your training program is what's realistic given your other commitments. If you'd like to work out three days a week, we could argue all day long about how it's optimal to space your workouts evenly across the week—Monday, Wednesday, and Friday, for instance—but if you're more likely to sustain your commitment by working out on Saturday, Sunday, and Monday, that's entirely fine! As is often said, the science is in the compliance. Better to diligently execute a decent plan than half-heartedly execute a perfect plan.

In most cases, if you are working out three or fewer days per week, full body workouts will make the most sense and give you the greatest return on the time you invest. This does not mean you will perform the exact same movements in each workout, but rather that each workout will include exercises addressing each of the fundamental movement patterns. The collective amount of work any given muscle will be able to perform will increase when you spread the work out across multiple days. That said, in cases where you might have training sessions on back- to-back days, it may make more sense to split your efforts in order to better promote recovery. For example, somebody who can only train on Saturday and Sunday may choose to perform squatting, pulling, and locomotion exercises on Saturday, and dedicate Sunday to hingeing, pushing, and core training. These sorts of training splits can also make sense for people who train more frequently; training the entire body five or six days a week might hinder recovery and make it difficult to truly challenge any given movement or muscle.

Splits might be oriented around movement patterns, such as having a "push" day, a "pull" day, and a "leg" day; some people treat squatting and lungeing movements as lower body "pushing" exercises and hinge-ing or other hamstring-dominant exercises as lower body "pulling" ex-ercises, such that the leg day could be subdivided into "lower push" and "lower pull" days in a four day weekly training split. Other programs organize the training week by focusing on specific muscle groups. One five-day per week example (I feel like every dedicated gym-goer I know has done some version of this at some point in their lives) might involve training the chest on Monday, the back on Tuesday, the shoulders on Wednesday, the legs on Thursday, and the arms and core on Friday. These days, I'm suspicious of people who only perform leg exercises once per week, but that's just me!

One way or the other, rest must be taken during the course of the training program. Ultimately, training presents a stress on the body from which it must recover. Training breaks the body down, and it's really through the recovery process— eating well, getting enough sleep, etc.—that we get bigger, faster, or stronger. Some people enjoy includ-ing some form of physical activity every day; there's nothing wrong with this, especially if some day's activities are of a much lower intensity or are actively focused on physical restoration. Indeed, rest and recovery aren't optimized by sitting on the couch sipping beer and eating na-chos; rest days can provide a wonderful opportunity to focus on mobil-ity work (such as stretching or massage), include extra walking or low-intensity cardiovascular work, or spend time on other things that facil-itate progress toward your fitness goals (I love the notion that Sunday's "workout" is grocery shopping and meal prep if the goal is fat loss—time well spent!).

Over the course of a training program, change must be made to continue making progress. During the program itself, it is more com-mon to change variables such as the weight being used (or speed in cardiovascular exercise), the volume performed (sets, reps, or duration) of a given exercise, or the amount of rest taken between exercise. Exercise selection may be varied within a program, but often is changed from one program to the next. Some of this depends on experience (a less experienced trainee will benefit from spending time getting more comfortable and skillful with a smaller variety of exercises) as well as personality (some people crave far more variety than others). Other variables such as training frequency or program emphasis (e.g. emphasizing strength development versus muscle growth) are generally adjusted in between programs, after any relevant assessments are performed. Ultimately, your body will adapt to stimuli and demands it experiences after enough exposure. According to a training principle known as progressive over load, you must continually challenge your body by shifting one of these variables (or more) if adaptation is to continue. Which variable(s) you choose depends on the goals you are trying to achieve and the progress that has been made. Indeed, the training program itself acts as a continual assessment process; every repetition, every set, every workout serves as a chance to evaluate progress, both objective and subjective. For a fat loss client, progress might be maintaining strength or cardiovascular stamina while losing weight (their relative strength has increased); for a strength-focused trainee, progress may simply be lifting more weight with the same perceived amount of effort. That said, the conclusion of one training program marks an important time to reflect upon the successes and/ or shortcomings of the work that has been performed and to use the data to make the best plan possible for the following block of training. If your goal is to run one mile in a faster time and you have made minimal progress but have succeeded in gaining muscle, this is valuable data! Certainly other lifestyle factors would need to be examined, but the training program can and should be revised in light of the assessment results.

Example Training Program

Below is an example of what a program could look like for somebody training three days per week. All of the workouts are full-body in nature and include a mixture of equipment; the strength exercises are organized into two circuits, each containing three exercises. This particular example may be appropriate for someone who has been training for a couple of months and does not have any substantial injuries or movement limitations, but adjustments could be easily made for someone who has less experience or needs to work around any sort of restriction. The cardiovascular training uses a variety of machines and incorporates different interval structures to allow development of capacity at different relative intensities.

3-DAY FULL-BODY PROGRAM
DAY 1

Warm-Up

A1) Kettlebell Goblet Squat (heels elevated on 10lb plates)
A2) Incline Dumbell Bench Press
A3) Lat Pulldown (palms facing toward each other)

B1) Side Lunge
B2) Farmers Carry
B3) Side Plank

C) Incline Treadmill Walk 15 Minutes at 70% effort

Cool-Down: foam rolling for legs and upper back, stretching for hipflexors and inner thighs

DAY 2

Warm-Up

A1) Dumbbell Bench Press

A2) One Arm Dumbbell Row

A3) Hip Thrust with Upper Back on Exercise Bench

B1) Crawl in Place

B2) Lying Hamstring Curl

B3) Suspension Strap Row

C) Rowing Machine 3 minutes work, 1 minute rest x4

Cool-Down: Deep Tissue Massage

DAY 3

Warm-Up

A1) Assisted Pull-Up

A2) Kettlebell Deadlift

A3) Seated Dumbbell Overhead Press

B1) Alternating Reverse Lunge

B2) Turkish Get-Up

B3) Kettlebell 1-Arm Farmer's Carry

C) Airbike or Stationary Bike 30 seconds work, 60 seconds rest x 8-10

Cool-down: 5 minutes of deep breathing/meditation, 10 minutes in steam room

Training for Successful Aging

Having established a practical framework for setting training goals and understanding how to structure your training routine accordingly, we will conclude with some specific thoughts on how to train to facilitate successful aging. By this we mean training in such a way as to maximize function, independence, and vitality as you get older. Eventually, performance and fitness goals are pursued in service of supporting general well-being (e.g., you might not want to irritate a cranky elbow just to do one more pull-up than the week before!). Regardless of your age, you can always train and improve your health and physical fitness; just make sure to start where you are, be patient, and progress appropriately. Examine your current routine for any sobvious gaps and consider training in a fashion that develops these attributes:

Strength, especially in the lower body and grip:

Basic strength training can do wonders for preserving lean body mass and preventing injury. Again, think of basic drills such as squats, dead-lifts, lunges, rows, pull-ups/lat pulldowns, push-ups/bench presses, and farmers carries (am I sounding like a broken record yet?). While age-related loss of muscle mass (known as sarcopenia) is inevitable, it can be greatly mitigated through resistance training, promoting general function as well as metabolic health. Gradual degradation of bone mass can eventually result in osteoporosis (often of particular concern for women) and, as a result, increased fragility - a fall that wouldn't phase a 12-year old in the slightest may well break the hip of an 89-year old.

Loading your body's tissues against the force of gravity may be one of the most important things you can do for injury prevention.

The lower body and grip may be especially important to prioritize for functioning independently through daily life. You need the strength to walk, go up and down stairs, and get up and down from the couch or toilet. Many of us have also seen commercials featuring an elderly person exclaiming, "Help, I've fallen and I can't get up!" While falls are extremely problematic as is, lacking the strength to recover and seek assistance can exacerbate an already dangerous situation. In addition to the fundamental movement patterns already outlined, training for successful aging should specifically include time spent getting up and down from the ground (with assistance, if needed). Grip strength will allow you to continue lifting heavy objects, open jars, and walk around holding your own groceries or luggage. Strength through the posterior chain (think hamstrings, glutes, and back) can also support maintaining a tall and upright posture. As alluded to earlier, strength is the master quality and will aid in maintaining joint mobility, muscular flexibility, and even power.

Coordination and Balance

We have spoken earlier about coordination and balance; in the context of training for healthy aging, these qualities can be especially important for safety. Training in a reactive fashion –that is, being presented with a relatively unpredictable stimulus and responding accordingly—can be tremendous for preserving reflexes. This can be as simple as playing a game of catch, or performing exercise in a manner similar to the game "Simon Says" (heaven forbid training should be so enjoyable as playing childhood games!). Enormous portions of the human brain are dedicated to the constant problem-solving process of receiving sensory information and responding with an appropriately coordinated movement. Indeed, exercise is generally regarded as one of the single most important things a person can do for maintaining cognitive health.

Balance exercises may be as simple as single-leg exercises such as lunges, single leg deadlifts, or slow marching, but again require substantial strength as well as coordination. Falling presents a great risk to physical health and well being; sadly, almost everyone can relate to knowing somebody whose health and well-being were greatly compromised after a bad fall, and in many cases with the elderly these falls seem to mark the beginning of a decline toward death. Training balance in conjunction with fundamental strength can be essential in preventing a fall outright; coordination and reflex training can aid in prevention as well, or at least in mitigating the damage of a fall (if you fall in the shower, I'd much rather have you catch yourself with your hands and hurt your wrists than bang your head off the tile).

Power

As alluded to earlier, power involves the rapid production or absorption of force. Remember that power is relative. For a firefighter, the expression of power might involve kicking down a door and sprinting up a flight of stairs; for a grandmother, this might mean quickly stepping out of the way as her grandchildren come barreling down the hall and threaten collision! Jumping out of the way of danger on time is expressing power by producing force; tripping on a crack in the sidewalk and rapidly catching all of your bodyweight on one leg is expressing power by absorbing force (again, we see that rapid force absorption - the ability to decelerate - is critical for fall prevention). Power is one of the qualities most readily lost with age, but - as with muscle loss - this decline can be greatly mitigated through training. Earlier we noted that power is essential to most sport activities such as running, jumping, throwing, and swinging (a bat, club, racket, etc.).

If you strive to feel vital and enjoy these activities into your later years, train accordingly!

Cardiovascular Endurance and Aerobic Capacity

Cardiovascular and metabolic diseases are two of the most common health issues many people face during their lives. Excess body fat, high blood pressure, insulin resistance, and abnormal elevation of cholesterol and/or triglycerides elevate the risk of heart attacks, diabetes, stroke, and other metabolic conditions. While exercise alone is often insufficient, and these issues should be addressed through a combination of lifestyle factors in conjunction with any necessary medical care, cardiovascular exercise can be a critical component of prevention or treatment. Moreover, successful aging is not merely the prevention of these disease states - our goal is to help you thrive in your later years! Cardiovascular training should be an essential part of any long-term training plan so that you may enjoy being physically active without being out of breath.

Joint Mobility & Muscular Flexibility

Gradual decreases in your available joint mobility and muscular flexibility eventual limit your movement options. As before, performing fundamental movements through full ranges of motion may be your single best bet for maintaining comfortable movement. Seek appropriate treatment, rehabilitation, and training for any injuries you may encounter along the journey of a life well-lived. Over time, you may find yourself dedicating extra time to physical recovery and restoration - massage, foam rolling, stretching, and mobility-focused exercise practices such as yoga or martial arts.

Pelvic Floor Function

Pelvic floor training may be treated as a particular branch of strength training, but merits particular discussion for those wishing to age gracefully.

While women may be more familiar with pelvic floor training through experience with pregnancy, childbirth, and menopause, both men and women can experience pelvic floor dysfunction as they age.

Resulting issues can include pain or discomfort, bladder and bowel issues, and sexual dysfunction. As per usual, pelvic floor issues should be addressed through a combination of medical treatment, when needed, alongside lifestyle factors including exercise, healthy nutrition, sleep, and stress management. Thankfully, exercise and physical activity in general can be highly beneficial for the strength and function of the pelvic floor.

Kegel exercises are specifically focused on strengthening the muscles of the pelvic floor - to perform these, try to replicate the sensation of stopping urination. Exercises specifically focused on strengthening nearby musculature (around the pelvis and hips) may also be of particular utility, though even low- to moderate-intensity physical activities such as walking can help. If you are currently experiencing pelvic floor issues, high intensity exercise, especially activities involving repeated impact forces, may be inappropriate; as always, make sure to consult with your physician regarding any medical issues that may impact your training.

CHAPTER SUMMARY:

PART 1

1. When establishing health and fitness goals, find clarity in the specific outcomes you'd like to achieve. One possible way to structure your goals is to make them SMART - specific, measurable, attainable, relevant, and time bound.

2. Determine whether your goals primarily relate to health, fitness, or body composition. These three categories largely overlap, but some goals may concentrate on one or two areas even at the possible expense of one of the others. The nature of your goal will be very important in shaping the choices you make with respect to exercise, nutrition, recovery, and other elements of daily life.

3. After clarifying your outcome goal, define your process goal(s) - specific behaviors and habits that are under your control. These behaviors, when executed consistently, should help you achieve your desired outcome goal. Pick 1-2 behaviors to focus on at a time in order to give yourself a high chance of achieving and sustaining success.

4. Periodically reassess your progress. Use both objective, quantitative measures that help you understand the relative progress you have made toward your outcome goal as well as subjective or qualitative assessments that might better reflect your experience of the change process. Also assess your consistency with the behavior(s) and habit(s) you are working on to best determine if they are sustainable and contributing positively to goal accomplishment. When you are ready, you can add additional layers in order to achieve additional progress. Use this continual

5. process of experimentation to learn about your preferences and what works well for you.

PART 2

1. Incorporate fundamental human movements into your training routine: squat, hinge, push, pull, core training, locomotion, breathing.

2. Begin training by establishing basic coordination, strength, and aerobic capacity while learning proper training technique. Develop and improve other physical qualities such as mobility, flexibility, balance, power, and endurance as needed depending on your specific training goals.

3. Arrange individual workouts to include a proper warm-up, power and strength training, cardiovascular work (aka energy systems development), and a cool down to begin the recovery process. Arrange the broader training program to fully train the entire body over the course of the training week (or some regular cycle of time); this can be done using full body workouts or training splits, which divide workouts by body part or types of movement.

4. Over time, progress variables such as the amount of weight used, volume (sets times repetitions), rest, training frequency, and exercise selection (using different exercises or veequipment - possibly, but not necessarily more complex). Which variables you change will be largely decided based on your goal.

5. Consider what it means to train in a way that supports long term well- being and allows you to thrive in your later years. Muscle mass and power are lost as part of the natural aging process, but losses of function and vitality can be greatly mitigated through training. Basic strength training, mobility and flexibility work,

and cardiovascular exercise will work wonders for maintaining independence and physical well-being, and may help to prevent injury and other common health conditions.

INDEX OF RECURRING SUBJECTS

Mind/Body/S pirit or (Res- piration) Breath:
27, 31, 47-8, 84-5, 129, 145, 158, 161, 171, 177-8, 188, 207, 217, 224-5, 229, 231, 236, 238-9

Mo- tion/Move- ment:
11, 14, 23-4. 26-9, 31-3, 60-1, 70, 78, 80, 95, 100, 107-9, 111, 123, 171, 198-9, 240, 243-6, 248-55, 258-63, 267, 274-80, 282-4, 286, 288-90, 293, 295, 297-9, 301

Neuro/n/Neu robehavioral/- endocrine/- genic/-lin- guistic/-logi- cal/-matrix/- muscular/- pathic/-plas- ticity/-psy- chology/-sci- ence or scien- tist/-tag/- transmitter:
11, 25-6, 29, 31, 46, 57, 69, 78, 84, 87, 89, 92, 96-8, 100-1, 104-7, 119, 129, 132-3, 150, 163, 165-6, 172, 174, 215, 243-4, 284, 289,

Nutrition:
13, 23-4, 29-31, 43, 47, 55-6, 60-1, 76, 114, 117-19, 130-6, 138-55, 188, 192, 195, 238, 263, 266-70, 288, 299-300

Pain:
22-3, 25-9, 31, 57, 63, 74, 81, 83-114, 133, 158, 161, 163, 165-6, 168-74, 178, 180-1, 191, 200, 205-6, 208, 216-7, 226-7, 234, 236-7, 240, 247, 264, 267, 274-5, 299